Devine Guidance

for Managing Key Attributes of a FDA-

Compliant Quality Management

System

Christopher Joseph Devine, Ph.D.

© 2013

Devine Guidance for Managing Key Attributes of a FDA-Compliant Quality Management System

Limit of Liability/Disclaimer of Warranty

The author has put forth his best effort in compiling the content of this book; however, no warranty with respect to material accuracy or completeness is made. Additionally, no warranty is made in regards to applying the recommendations made in this book to any business structure or environment. The advice and recommendations provided within this book may not be suitable for all business structures or environments. Businesses should consult regulatory, quality, and/or legal professionals prior to deciding on the appropriateness of advice and recommendations made within this book. The author shall not be held liable for loss of profit or other commercial damages resulting in the employment of recommendations made within this book including; special, incidental, consequential, or other damages.

ISBN-13: 978-1500209995

ISBN-10: 1500209996

About the Author

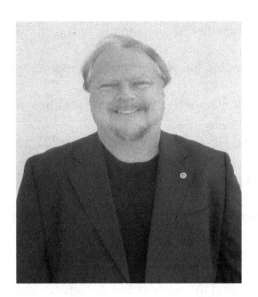

Dr. Christopher Joseph Devine

Dr. Christopher Joseph Devine, Ph.D. is the President of Devine Guidance International, a consulting firm specializing in providing solutions for regulatory compliance, quality, supplier management, and supply-chain issues facing the medical device industry. Additionally, Dr. Devine is the author of Devine Guidance, a weekly blog focusing on the understanding of regulations mandated by the FDA and other regulatory bodies; and published by the Medical Device Summit, an *e*-magazine. Furthermore, Dr. Devine is a member of the editorial board of the Medical Device Summit. Dr. Devine has 35-years of experience in quality assurance, regulatory affairs, and program management. He is a senior member of the American Society of Quality (ASQ), a member of Regulatory Affairs Professionals Society (RAPS), a member of the Project Management Institute (PMI), a member of the Society of Manufacturing Engineers (SME), and resides on several technical advisory boards. Dr. Devine received his doctorate from Northcentral University, with his doctoral dissertation entitled, "Exploring the Effectiveness of Defensive-Receiving Inspection for Medical Device Manufacturers: A Mixed-Method Study." Dr. Devine also holds a graduate degree in organizational management (MAOM) and an undergraduate degree business management (BSBM). Prior to Dr. Devine's commercial career he served proudly as a member of the United States Marine Corps.

Dedication

To my family, especially my wife Connie, and my kids Kelly, Erin, and Travis, for their patience with me while spending long hours on the computer; to Elijah Christopher, my grandson, congratulations on your alligator wresting abilities; to my son-in-law Gilberto – welcome to the family and Go A's; to my dear and trusted friend Dr. Ron Allen who mentored and reminded me that once I received my doctorate, I was obligated to write (book number five my friend); to my dear friend Jim Twitchell (Twitch) thank you for the drinking and thinking sessions; to my dear friend Randy (Hoyt) Smith, thank you for the long hours on the phone and the support and the understanding of the "FYR" concept; to my dear friend Brian Ludovico, Rayshon Payne, and my friends at TUV-R – thank you for your ongoing support; to Roberta Goode and Jeremy Cortese (GCI) thank you for the opportunities; to my dear friends at Sensus Healthcare (Kal Fishman, Joseph Sardano, and Michael Sardano) – the SRT-100 Vision Radiotherapy System rocks, to my old friend Dennis Wong – thank you for the referrals, to my friend David Lamb – good luck in your new endeavor; to my friend Rey Rara – keep the faith my friend, to my oldest and dearest friend Jace Smith, we made it out the hood my friend; to my good friend and most excellent guitar player "Mad Mike" Rosenboom – keep rock'n out man; to the RA Team at BIOMET 3i (Jackie Hughes, Anne Mulvihill, Jean Shen, Laura HoShue, and Mark Mashburn) – there is light at the end of the tunnel and it is not a train coming the other way down the tracks; to some of my favorite readers Frank Pokrop and John Upham – Thank You; and finally to my parents, Joseph T. & Dorothy L. Devine, although they have passed, they would be proud of Dr. D's accomplishments.

Acknowledgements

First and foremost, I want to thank Rick and Beth Biros, Mark Spector, Tom Maeder, and the entire staff of the Medical Device Summit. They continue to give me the opportunity to publish my work in a weekly forum (Devine Guidance) in this fabulous on-line industry magazine. I would also like to recognize Sangita Viswanathan, the editor of the Medical Device Summit, for her painstaking review and editing of my weekly articles. Finally, to the readers of Devine Guidance; without your ongoing patronage there would be no Devine Guidance. Yes, the doctor knows that most of you like me, some of you despise me, and a few of you have no opinion. For those of you with no opinion, you truly frighten Dr. D, as all quality and regulatory professionals should have an opinion.

Introduction

The purpose of Dr. D's fifth book is to provide the readers some additional insight into not only entering devices into the US market place but actually keeping them there. The doctor actually loves the US device market place because the FDA regulations are relatively static. Now that doesn't mean the FDA does not adopt and change to an increasingly dynamic medical device environment in the United States. However, it does mean that FDA is careful when implementing changes to regulatory and statutory requirements versus the EU where the directives change just for the sake of change. Another point Dr. D is compelled to make is that once devices are cleared and or approved (depending on regulatory pathway), they will remain available on the US market, providing they remain safe and effective; however, in Europe not so much. In fact, the notified bodies have turned reviewing the renewal of Class III device applications (design dossiers) into a profit center as design examination certificates (licenses) require renewal every three to five years, depending on the notified body. In fact notified bodies charge for managing your certificates. Seriously? You pay them for managing paper? Considering all of the upcoming changes proposed in the EU, including the rescript of the MDD into a regulation, working in the US device market is actually refreshing and predictable. Before you even ask, yes notified bodies have the authority to extend certificates for one certification period but seldom if ever do so. Why - Because it is all about the money baby. Anyway, enough of the doctor digressing and back to the topic at hand entering and keeping devices in the US market place. Just as a point of reference, the doctor has taken the opportunity to make some references to the EU so the readers come away with a fundamental understanding of some of the differences between

the United States and Europe. I hope you find value in Dr. D's fifth book and as always,

if you have questions please feel free to contact the doctor at

chris.devine@devineguidanceinternational.com. Enjoy the book!

Devine Guidance for Managing Key Attributes of a FDA-Compliant Quality Management System

Table of Contents

Devine Guidance for Managing Key Attributes of a FDA-Compliant Quality Management System

Devine Guidance the Rules

Dr. D's Rules

Ever since Dr. D's childhood, I have always had a major aversion to rules of any kind. After all, rules are established so creative folks can bend or break them. Unfortunately, bending or breaking rules in the medical device industry can result in device manufacturers ending up in regulatory purgatory or even worse. In fact, the conveyors of the rules can really unload some serious hurt on device manufacturers not willing to adhere to their rules or intentionally take liberties in regards to their rules. That being said, the doctor has created a set of rules that should keep device organizations on the straight and narrow path of compliance. As you will quickly see, these rules are premised on one very simple concept, "common sense." Enjoy.

- Rule #1 - Compliance to regulations is not optional; compliance is mandatory and dictated by law.

- Rule #2 - Measuring and monitoring equipment shall be calibrated, maintained, and traceable back to a recognized standard, e.g. NIST.

- Rule #3 - Document the results of all events in writing, because if it is not documented, in writing, the event did not occur.

- Rule #4 – The FDA conducts inspections for the purpose of collecting evidence, should legal action be required; while your notified body (*remember they work for you*) conduct audits. Treat each visit accordingly.

- Rule #5 – All investigations, CAPAs, Response Required SCARs, product failures, audit findings, etc. requires root-cause analysis and follow-up for effectiveness of the actions pursued.

- Rule #6 – All procedures, work instructions, drawings, specifications, etc. must be written, well-documented, and controlled within a defined document control system (No napkin drawings, please).

- Rule #7 – Make sure all changes, design, process, supplier, etc. are processed through the appropriate level of verification and/or validation.

- Rule #8 – Clearly mark and segregate all non-conforming material, preferably under lock and key.

- Rule #9 – Management review is an important tool employed to gage the effectiveness of your entire organization, not just quality; so ensure all of the metrics employed to monitor your business are included into the review.

- Rule #10 – Effective design control is not an option, it is a salient requirement.

- Rule #11 – Never have your quality or regulatory organizations report into manufacturing operations, i.e., the separation of church and state rule.

- Rule #12 – Traceability is required from start to finish for everything, i.e., production, process validation, design validation, aging studies, etc.

- Rule #13 – When in doubt, read the appropriate regulation or Directive, contact your notified body, talk with your quality organization or regulatory organization, and finally yet importantly, ask for Devine Guidance.

- Rule #14 – You do not have to share the results or content of internal audits, supplier audits, or management reviews with the FDA; however, you must provide evidence that this activities are occurring.

- Rule #15 - Post-market surveillance is an important activity. Please ensure all customer complaints are actively logged, investigated to root-cause (if possible), and a response returned to the complaining organization.

- Rule #16 - Responses to MDRs and vigilance reports should be deemed mission critical. If an organization builds a documented history of late reporting of MDRs and vigilance reports, they can expect a visit from their friends from the agency and the Competent Authorities.

- Rule #17 – Do not affix the CE Marking of Conformity to product until your notified body grants permission, in writing.

- Rule #18 – The relationship with the notified body should be treated like a marriage; hopefully, a good one.

- Rule #19 – Believe what you will, but the IVDD, MDD, and AIMDD are law in the European Union.

- Rule #20 – Member States retain the legal write to have labeling (Instructions for Use and product labels) in their native tongue.

- Rule #21 – Technical Files and Design Dossiers are dynamic documents that must be kept current.

- Rule #22 – Use of Harmonized Standards, although not mandated by law, is strongly recommended.

- Rule # 23 – Make sure the Chief Jailable Officer (CJO) signs all Declarations of Conformity (DoC). Note: for Japan the CJO becomes the Chief Impalable Officer (CIO) that will fall onto a sword versus wearing an orange jumpsuit.

"If Dr. D's rules do not fit your application, you can always establish your own!"

Establishment Registration

Establishment Registration

If your organization has already bellied up to the FDA bar and paid the $2,575 (2013) bar tab to the FDA; and listed your medical devices through the FDA Unified Registration and Listing System (FURLS); then no worries, you are in compliance with 21 CFR, Part 807 (from an establishment registration perspective). For those of you working for organizations that have failed to register as an establishment, Dr. D has provided a "*myriad*" (look-it-up) of excuses you can give to the FDA when they magically appear on your facility's door step.

- We could not afford the registration fee.

- We did not think our product is a medical device.

- We are just a contract manufacturer.

- We only import and export medical devices.

- We are not a US-based device manufacturer.

- We only sterilize devices.

- We like to push the limit and ignore laws.

- What's Part 807?

- Who is FDA?

Unfortunately, every one of the responses equates to poking a stick into the eye of a sleeping bear. When running from a ticked-off bear one does not have to be the fastest runner; just do not be the slowest. However, with the FDA, there is no running, only pain for failing to register as an establishment and list the medical devices you manufacturer, assemble, sterilized, distribute, etc.

Devine Guidance for Managing Key Attributes of a FDA-Compliant Quality Management System

For those of you living in a cave or oblivious to the ongoing change in the regulatory environment in the United States, on August 2, 2012, the FDA sent an open letter to the medical device industry advising the industry of significant changes to the establishment registration process. The changes to establishment registration went into effect on October 1, 2012. As a result of the changes to the establishment registration process, Title 21 CFR, Part 807 was revised. On another note; it sure would be nice if the agency updated their web site and posted the most current version of part 807. The doctor just checked and the April 1, 2012 version is still posted. That being said, Dr. D would think that with all of this additional revenue being paid into FDA as a result of expanding the establishment registration field, they could afford to update their website.

What the doctor truly finds amazing there are organizations out there that are now required to register but are failing to do so. For example, if you are a machine shop manufacturing bone screws for the orthopedics industry and you are the last ones touching the screws, you are a contract manufacturer and need to register. If you are operating an ethylene oxide sterilization facility in Timbuktu and the sterilized finish device eventually make their way into the US device market, you must register. In short, $2575 (2013) is the price of admission to play in the US medical device industry sandbox. Some of the salient changes to the establishment registration process are:

- If your organization is required to register as an establishment, then you must pay to play, so if you have not already done so, write that check for $2575.

- Device manufacturers (foreign and domestic) are required to register with FDA, pay the man.

- Contract manufacturers (foreign and domestic) are required to register with FDA, pay the man.

- Contract sterilizers (foreign and domestic) are required to register with FDA, pay the man.

- Device manufacturers are required to list their products with FDA through the use of FURLS.

- Contract manufacturers and sterilizers are required to list the products they manufacturer and sterilize, including the medical device they are performing the work for using FURLS.

- In fact, Devices are now required to be listed by the: (a) manufacturer; (b) specification developer; (c) device re-processors; (d) remanufacturers; (e) device re-packers; and (f) device re-labelers; before listing by foreign exporters; contract manufacturers, or contract sterilizers.

Takeaways

For this chapter, the doctor will leave the readers with just one pearl of wisdom. If you have not registered with FDA as an establishment and your organization meets the requirements delineated within Part 807, then what is stopping you? There is no time like the present to write the $2575 (2013 Fee) check to the agency. Failure to register when required to do so, can result in the agency opening a can of regulatory whoop-ass resulting in varying degrees of pain. Can you say the FDA has told us to stop shipping product? Can you say interruption of the revenue stream?

"Establishment registration is not an option so stop making excuses and register!"

Class I Devices

Class I Devices

Some of the sweetest words medical device manufacturers like to hear are: "Class I Exempt." Simply put, no pre-market application, a.k.a., 510(k) submission is required to market the device. However, device manufacturers are still required to register their establishment with FDA, pay the $2,575 (FY 2013), and list their device(s) using the FDA Unified Registration and Listing System (FURLS). For those readers not familiar with the agency's classification system, the FDA employs three classifications of devices premised on risk, with Class I being the lowest risk and Class III being the highest risk. Dr. D does not typically employ an *"effusive"* (look-it-up) style of writing; however, the doctor cannot place enough emphasis on understanding the regulatory pathways associated with placing finished medical devices on the U.S. market. Enjoy.

Class I Devices

The doctor has taken the liberty of extracting what the FDA considers requirements for a Class I device from the agency's website.

> *FDA has exempted almost all class I devices (with the exception of Reserved Device) from the premarket notification requirement, including those devices that were exempted by final regulation published in the Federal Registers of December 7, 1994, and January 16, 1996. Some 510(k) exemptions annotated with "\#\" are with certain limitations as noted in the footnotes. It is important to confirm the exempt status and any limitations that apply with 21 CFR Parts 862-892. Limitations of device exemptions are covered under 21 CFR xxx.9, where xxx refers to Parts 862-892.*

> *If a manufacturer's device falls into a generic category of exempted class I devices as defined in 21 CFR Parts 862-892, a premarket notification application and FDA clearance is not required before marketing the device in the U.S. However, these manufacturers are required to register their establishment and list the generic category or classification name. Registration and listing information is submitted by using FDA's Unified Registration and Listing System (FURLS)/ Device Registration and Listing Module (DRLM) at:*

http://www.fda.gov/MedicalDevices/DeviceRegulationandGuidance/HowtoMarke tYourDevice/RegistrationandListing/ucm053185.htm[9]

IMPORTANT NOTE: *Only the class I devices with an asterisk (*) are also exempted from the GMP regulation, except for general requirements concerning records (820.180) and complaint files (820.198),* ***as long as the device is* not *labeled or otherwise represented as* sterile.**

So what does the FDA require for Class I devices from a Quality System regulation (QSR) standpoint? Typically, the term "*General Controls*" is associated with Class I devices. General controls consist of:

- Registering the medical device manufacturing establishment with the FDA;

- Listing devices with FDA using FURLS;

- Manufacturing devices in accordance with FDA Good Manufacturing Practices (GMP), with a focus on quality control, complaint handling, and record keeping; and

- Labeling medical devices to provide explicit instructions for use (IFU), including warning statements, to ensure the safe and effective use of medical devices in their intended use.

For the regular readers of Dr. D's fine prose on quality and regulatory compliance, I am sure you are wondering why the doctor has not thrown in one of his smart-alecky remarks. Here cones one. It is incumbent upon the Chief Jailable Officer (CJO) to ensure all devices, under his or her domain, are appropriately cleared and listed in FURLS. Hey CJO, this is not rocket science, it is the law. The doctor has been led to believe the price of orange jumpsuits has skyrocketed so compliance with QSR appears to be a viable option. Besides, no device manufacturer wants the FDA to back-up the proverbial turnip truck and hall away a truck full of adulterated/misbranded devices.

Takeaways

For this chapter's guidance, the doctor will leave the readers with just one takeaway. Although the regulatory burden is greatly reduced for Class I devices, in the eyes of FDA it is still a medical device. Manufacturers of Class I devices are still required to register their establishment with FDA, list their device(s) in the FURLS, and maintain general controls.

"Regardless of device classification, you must list all devices using FURLS!"

Class II Devices

Class II Devices

As stated in the previous chapter, the FDA premises device classification based on risk. Low-risk devices are Class I and high-risk devices are Class III. The doctor is going to assume that this not earth-shattering news for the masses. So if Class I is low-risk and Class III is high-risk, then just maybe Class II is medium-risk (well sort of). That is one way to look at it. For starters, similar to Class I devices, manufacturers of Class II devices are required to register with FDA as an establishment in accordance with 21 CFR, Part 807. By the way did Dr. D mention you have to pay Uncle Sam $2,575 (for 2013) to register as an establishment with FDA? Additionally, all Class II devices, once cleared by the FDA, must be listed in the FDA User and Registration Listing System (FURLS). So what does cleared device mean Dr. D? Read on my dear readers (next section) and the doctor will provide some insight into cleared devices. The good news is Dr. D has never been categorized as being "*labile*" (look-it-up) just a little "*insolent*" (look-it-up) and tenacious when on the pulpit pontificating about compliance. Enjoy.

Class II Devices

Well if you made it this far, the doctor is going to climb out on a limb and assume you are still interested in this chapter's guidance. If you are continuing to read because Dr. D's fine proses irritate you, that is ok too, Dr. D loves you man! With a few minor exceptions, the regulatory path to obtain clearance from the FDA, for a Class II device, is through the submission of a well-written 510(k) that adheres to FDA guidelines delineated within 21 CFR, Part 807. The 510(k) is premised on their being a predicate device that has previously blazed the regulatory path and obtained FDA clearance.

Remember for the 510(k), the submitter must list a predicate device (list one predicate, and if necessary multiple reference devices). The underlying concept of the 510(k) is to establish substantial equivalence with the claimed predicate.

There are 21 Sections associated with a 510(k). There is a good chance, not all sections may be applicable for your 510(k). If not all of the sections apply, **do not list N/A and stop.** The prudent path is to list the section as Not Applicable and provide a brief paragraph explaining why a section is not applicable. If the 510(k) is deemed incomplete, the FDA will reward the device manufacturer with a "Refusal to Accept Letter."

Similar to establishment registration fees, you must pay Uncle Sam for an FDA review of the 510(k). For FY 2013, the review fee for a 510(k) is $4,960 for a large business and $2,480 for a small business (revenue ≤ $100 million). As of December 31st of 2012, you must file one copy of the 510(k) electronically. By the way, have fun with the e-filing system as the software is not user friendly. If it is your first time, allocate a couple of days, especially if your 510(k) is enormous.

Once you have filed the 510(k), the fun begins. If the FDA accepts the submission, the review clock starts ticking; tic, tic, tic, etc. If a device manufacturer does not hear from FDA after 90-days of a 510(k)'s initial submission, the manufacturer can file a Form FDA 3541 and ask for status. Just a quick note, at last glance the FDA was averaging approximately 141 days for each 510(k) review, so practicing patience really becomes a necessary virtue. For those of you that were not particularly clear with your submission or providing the necessary supporting documentation, now comes the endless barrage of questions from the reviewer. The doctor's experience is that if you receive fewer than ½ dozen questions, then pat yourself on the back, you have done well; and seven or more, not so much. The good news is that at the end of the entire process is a letter from the FDA notifying your organization that the device(s) covered by the 510(k) is/are cleared to market in the United States; henceforth the term "***cleared device***."

If you have failed to convince the agency that your device is substantially equivalent to the claimed predicate, there is a path for appeal through the use of the FDA appeals process and the use of an ombudsman (note process changed on May 17, 2013). Good luck with that. Just remember, it could always be worse, the FDA could ask for clinical data to support the submission. If that happens, cha-ching the price of admission to the U. S. device market place has just increased.

Takeaways

The doctor will leave the readers with three takeaways from this chapter's guidance. One – make sure the predicate device you select for the 510(k) process is actually an equivalent device. Two – make sure the 510(k) is complete. Dr. D always recommends placing the checklist employed by the FDA reviewers in the front of the 510(k) so the reviewer can easily ascertain that the submission contains all of the required elements. Three – if you receive questions from the reviewer, provide the requested clarification or information quickly. If you do not want your 510(k) sitting on the reviewer's desk collecting dust, a punctual response should be deemed mission critical.

"Class II devices require a submission of a 510(k) to FDA and formal FDA clearance prior to marketing these devices in the United States!"

Class III Devices

Class III Devices

Can you say Pre-market Approval (PMA)? Good for you, but do you know what the PMA process entails? If so, golf clap and a hearty "good for you." You can read this chapter's guidance for its entertainment value. For those readers wishing to learn just a tad-bit more about the FDA's PMA process; please continue with the reading of this chapter's guidance. Dr. D will attempt to teach, enlighten, and hopefully entertain you in the process. If your chief Jailable officer (CJO) believes that short-cuts are always available when pursuing a PMA, the doctor just purchased the new eastern span of the Bay Bridge and would like to sell it. The doctor will be the first one to tell colleges that the FDA's approval process for Class III device can be perceived as a *"sinuous"* (look-it-up) path. This is especially true if the FDA has concerns over the pallet full of data an organization has submitted as their PMA.

Class III Devices

Similar to Class I and Class II device, device manufacturers are required to register with FDA as an establishment in accordance with 21 CFR, Part 807; and all Class III devices are required to be listed in the FDA User and Registration Listing System (FURLS). However, the regulatory pathway for a Class III device is considerably more precarious. For starters, Dr. D recommends that you read 21 CFR, Part 814 as this document will dive into the PMA application process and shed light on FDA's responsibility under the regulation. Class III devices are considered high risk devices. The agency's PMA process is a scientific and regulatory process designed to review the safety and efficacy of Class III medical devices. This is real rocket science, right?

According to FDA;

> **"Class III** *devices usually sustain or support life, are implanted, or present potential unreasonable risk of illness or injury. They have the toughest regulatory controls. Most of these devices require Premarket Approval because general and special controls alone cannot reasonably assure their safety and effectiveness."*

The regulations allow for FDA to take 180-days for the PMA review process. Remember the bridge Dr. D has for sale, well if you believe the 180-day review process is a realistic timeframe, the doctor is also selling the Brooklyn Bridge too! Dr. D believes you should allocate at least 12-months for the agency's review process. Yes, the sales and marketing folks are going to scream about time to market, but hey we are talking about Class III devices and not tongue suppressors. As for the PMA application process, it is strongly recommend that you confer with the agency in advance. Number one, the FDA will be better prepared to commence with the PMA review process associated with your organization's submission; and number two, it will set the initial expectations in regards to the review process. Section 814.20 delineates the PMA application process. As a minimum, the application will need to contain (as applicable):

- Applicant name and address;

- Table of contents;

- Product summary containing: (a) indications for use; (b) device description; (c) alternative practices and procedures; (d) marketing history; (e) summary of clinical and non-clinical studies; and (f) conclusions drawn from the studies.

- A detailed description of: (a) device; (b) functional components/ingredients; (c) device properties; (d) theory of operation; and (e) manufacturing methods;

- References to claimed standards;

- Technical sections including: (a) results of nonclinical laboratory testing; (b) biological compatibility testing; (c) aging studies; (d) package testing, etc.

- Compliance statement for studies stating that the studies were performed in accordance with Part 812 or Part 813 (for example);

- Rationale for when clinical data comes from just one investigation site;

- Bibliography of published reports;

- Samples of the device, if requested by FDA;

- Copies of proposed device labeling;

- Environmental assessment;

- Financial certification and disclosure statement;

- Other information requested by FDA; and finally,

- **Do not forget to sign the application!**

Please remember that patience truly is a virtue when navigating the FDA's PMA process. Chances are good that there will be questions coming from FDA. In fact, expect a boatload of questions. If the clinical trials were mismanaged or the clinical data requires too much manipulation to support product safety and efficacy, i.e., too much time spending trying to normalize the statistical data sets; then expect a long and *"arduous"* (look-it-up) path.

Finally, did the doctor mention that the review fees for PMAs are not cheap? For FY 2013 the fee for a PMA is $248,000 ($62,000 for small businesses with revenue less than $100 million). Folks, the price tag alone should be reason enough to ensure the PMA is bullet proof prior to submitting the pallet full of documentation to FDA.

Takeaways

For this chapter's guidance the doctor will provide the readers with just one takeaway, be meticulous and thorough in the preparation of the PMA. The FDA

considers PMA devices high risk, and as such, expect an entirely new level of detail

versus the 510(k) process. Make sure all of the supporting data, reports, written rational

etc. are included as part of the submission process; and make sure there is **just one point

of contact** to interface with FDA.

"Versus a Class II device, the regulatory pathway for a Class III device is considerably more precarious!"

The FDA's Inspection Process

The FDA's Inspection Process

Can you say; "Can I please see the FDA Form 482?" Let Dr. D ask a more basic question, do you know the actual purpose of a Form 482? The Form 482 is the vehicle employed by FDA to announce their presence for an establishment inspection in the United States. The Notice of Inspection form will be presented by the investigator(s), along with their credentials when they show up on your door step for a cup of coffee and an inspection. From the very second the investigator enters into a medical device manufacturer's lobby, an escort should accompany this individual at all times, including trips to the use the restroom. Dr. D strongly suggests that all device manufacturers have a scripted SOP for managing agency inspections and all other kinds of regulatory visits, including notified body audits. Remember, during the "*incipient*" (look-it-up) stages of an FDA establishment inspection the tone is set for the entire inspection. It is important that professionalism be exuded by all employees during the inspection. It is imperative that all employees are reminded that FDA is on-site and random gossip could be the kiss of regulatory death during an inspection. That being said, Dr. D hopes you enjoy this chapter's guidance.

For starters, the FDA is tasked with providing regulatory oversight to well-over 150,000 domestic establishments (food, drug, medical devices, biologics, dietary supplements, etc.). For the medical device industry, the number of establishments has increased to more than 40,000 domestic establishments. Considering the significant number of establishments requiring FDA oversight, Dr. D hopes the readers can come to the quick conclusion that establishments manufacturing high-risk medical devices, a.k.a., Class III – PMA devices, have the highest priority when it comes to agency inspections.

For the readers of DG that are tasked with manufacturing Class I devices, relax – but not too much. The FDA's authority to perform establishment inspections comes directly from the Act.

Food, Drug and Cosmetic Act 21 USC §374

> *"704(a)(l): For purposes of enforcement of this Act, officers or employees duly designated by the Secretary, upon presenting appropriate credentials and a written notice to the O\\1ler, operator, or agent in charge, are authorized (A) to enter, at reasonable times, any factory, warehouse, or establishment in which food, drugs, devices, or cosmetics are manufactured, processed, packed, or held, for introduction into interstate commerce or after such introduction, or to enter any vehicle being used to transport or hold such food, drugs, devices, or cosmetics in interstate commerce; and (B) to inspect, at reasonable times and within reasonable limits and in a reasonable manner, such factory, warehouse, establishment, or vehicle and all pertinent equipment, finished and unfinished materials, containers, and labeling therein... "*

QSIT

For those of you not familiar with the acronym QSIT, it represents the FDA's approach to establishment inspections; Quality System Inspection Technique. In short, FDA has an inspection script that they are trained and adhere to in support of the inspection process. As the doctor is sure most of the readers are aware, the FDA can announce a planned inspection, in advance, or just show up at the front door unannounced. Regardless the agency will be well-prepared for the inspection, so it is critical that all medical device manufacturers are always in a state of compliance and ready to support an inspection. From an agency perspective, the inspection process can be broken down into six parts:

- Preparing for an inspection;

- Initiating the inspection;

- Performing the inspection;

- Collecting and documenting objective evidence;

- Closing the inspection; and

- Issuing the inspection report and follow-up actions.

Preparing for an Inspection

As previously stated, agency inspections (domestic) will be either announced or unannounced. Regardless, your job as a medical device quality and/or regulatory professional is to always have your organization prepared for such a visit. Prior to the agency's visit, the assigned investigator(s) will: (a) review your organization's compliance history; (b) review applicable guidance documents; (c) obtain a listing of all products cleared and approved for entry into the US market; (d) review inspection guidelines; and (e) prepare an inspection tool kit. Simply stated, the FDA will be prepared so device manufacturers should be at least equally prepared. As previously stated, Dr. D strongly recommends the scripting of a procedure that provides guidance for your organization for FDA inspections. In fact, a procedure should be scripted to cover all regulatory inspections and notified body audits. Additionally, every-single employee from the CEO down to the janitor needs to be trained to ensure the entire organization properly conducts themselves during an FDA inspection. If your organization has a few malcontents, lock these folks up in the janitor's closet.

Initiating the Inspection

Regardless of the inspection being announced or unannounced, the process commences when the investigator(s) arrive in the lobby. They will announce themselves and ask for the "most responsible person" or as Dr. D likes to say: "Chief Jailable Officer" CJO. The FDA will present their credentials and issue the Form 482 "Notice of Inspection." Once the investigator(s) enter the building, they should be escorted to a conference room that will be dedicated to the inspection. As part of the introductions, the investigator(s) will discuss the parameters of the inspection with the management team. Under **_no circumstances_** should FDA be permitted to travel through the facility without an escort that has been properly trained. Additionally, a competent individual should be identified as the inspection scribe. This individual or group of individuals will be tasked with the recording of the inspection minutes.

Performing the Inspection

During the inspection process the investigator(s) will ask for a ton of documentation to review. Dr. D strongly suggests establishing a backroom to ensure all documentation is adequately reviewed before placing it in front of the investigator(s). Yes, in a perfect world such a secondary review would not be necessary; however, Mr. Murphy is alive and well in the medical device industry.

Furthermore, as the inspection begins all SOPs given to the investigator(s) to review should be logged. In fact, Dr. D strongly recommends making two copies: (a) one for the FDA; and (b) a retain copy for the device manufacturer's records. During the inspection, the investigator(s) will ask for a plant tour and will probably want to visit critical manufacturing areas. Please ensure that any FDA facing person does not suffer from that dreadful disease known as; *__The deer in the headlights disease.__* In fact, all answers made to the investigator(s) should be short, sweet, and to the point. Sometimes a simple yes or no will do. Remember to remind all personnel that if they do not have an answer to an investigator's question, they should state; "I do not know but will get the answer and get back to you." Finally, make sure your organization's Subject Matter Experts (SME) only respond to questions pertaining to their functional areas of expertise.

Collecting and Documenting Objective Evidence

Please keep in mind the fundamental purpose of an agency inspection is to collect objective evidence of compliance or non-compliance. As part of the inspection, the investigator(s) will ask to see records that support compliance and may even ask for product samples. If product samples are requested, ensure that the entire transaction is properly documented, including a packing slip. It is an acceptable practice to ask the FDA to pay for sample devices collected during an inspection. The salient point that needs to be driven home is that the evidence collected can be used against the device manufacturer if the agency determines additional regulatory action is required. Unlike a notified body audit, evidence collected by the FDA can be admissible in the federal courts as evidence in a criminal case; or during the negotiation of a consent decree.

Closing the Inspection

During the inspection closeout, the FDA will discuss the results of the inspection and observations noted with the management team. One thing to keep in mind, this is not the forum to vehemently argue the validity of an observation. In fact, if the observation is minor the best practice is to acknowledge the observation and promise to correct the observation so the investigator(s) can annotate onto the Form 483 "Inspectional Observations" the commitment by management to correct. Finally, if the FDA is walking away with samples, they will leave you with a Form 484 "Receipt of Samples." From an inspection standpoint, it does not get much easier: (a) Form 482 - Notice of Inspection; (b) Form 483 – Inspectional Observations; and (c) Form 484 – Receipt of Samples.

Issuing the Inspection Report and Follow-up Actions

The last step performed by the investigator(s) is the writing of the Establishment Inspection Report (EIR). The EIR will be a summary of the inspection and a compilation of noted inspectional observations. Depending on the outcome of the inspection, the FDA can pursue additional regulatory action. On the positive side if a medical device establishment receives no Form 483 observations or a small number of minor observations, a voluntary compliance statement made by the establishment and the formal correction of the observations is all that is required. However, if a firm promises to correct observations and during the next agency inspection it is noted that the previous observation(s) were not corrected or the correction deemed ineffective, then receipt of a warning letter can be expected. Other regulatory tools the agency can employ to drive compliance are:

- Follow-up inspections;

- Regulatory meetings;

- Warning letters;

- Product seizures;

- Product injunctions;

- Consent decrees; and

- Criminal and civil penalties.

Takeaways

For this chapter's guidance, the doctor will leave the readers with five takeaways. *One* – a medical device manufacturer's best defense during an FDA inspection is to always be in compliance with the quality system regulation and all applicable parts of the regulation. *Two* – device manufacturers should always have a written procedure that delineates all of the organization's requirements for entertaining a regulatory inspection. *Three* – never place an individual suffering from the dreaded "deer in the headlights disease" in front of the FDA. *Four* – if the CJO does not look good in an orange jumpsuit with stainless-steel bracelets, then compliance will always be this individual's best friend. *Five* – lock all malcontents in the broom closet (just kidding – just keep them away from FDA).

Ensure that any FDA facing person does not suffer from that dreadful disease known as; "The deer in the headlights disease!"

So You Received a Form 483 from FDA, Deal with it!

So You Received a 483 from FDA, Deal with it!

The FDA has just finished an inspection and the results were not as stellar as your organization expected. In fact, the investigator has decided to leave your organization with a little gem, a Form 483 with multiple inspectional observations. Deal with it! The good news is you do not have to respond to the 483. The bad news is that if you fail to respond, the FDA will send your organization another little gift, a warning letter. So what is the Chief Jailable Officer (CJO) to do? Frankly, the CJO can start by asking the investigator about the observations noted and ensure the basis for the observations is understood. The CJO can disagree with an observation; however, vehemently arguing with the investigator, sheading real tears, holding one's breath, screaming, or dropping to the floor and throwing a temper tantrum is not going to work. Frankly, if the 483 is for one or two minor issues, even if you disagree, just bite the bullet and fix the perceived issue. In any event, if the CJO agrees with the observations, ensure the "promise to correct" annotation is noted on the Form 483. Remember, the agency is not trying to "*thimblerig*" (look-it-up) device manufacturers into signing the 483.

Just Respond Baby

As the doctor stated, begin by understanding the basis for the Form 483 observations. Not wanting to state the obvious but obliged to do so, Dr. D believes that the offending organization just might have a compliance issue, if multiple observations are noted. If the organization is blessed with several 483 observations, the agency just might say the heck with it, and move to warning letter. Don't laugh, it happens and happens more frequently than most CJO's care to admit. From an agency perspective, they issue 483s when an inspector determines an organization has failed to comply with a specific part of the code delineated under the Act, typically, 21 CFR, Part 820 (the Quality System Regulation). FDA employs the 483 as a vehicle to ensure organizations quickly and promptly correct noted observations. In wrestling terms, it is what is called a choke hold. As Dr. D has already alluded to, a response is not mandated by law; however, the agency has the ability to unleash a whole lot of pain for organizations that choose not to comply with the request for correction. Trust the doctor when I say, "If the agency is not happy with your organization's response to the 483, your organization is not going to be happy when they receive the warning letter." Remember, "Warning letters equate to pain!" Fail to respond to the warning letter, and the Department of Justice and the federal courts will be in the offending device manufacturer's future. CJO's do not have to be clairvoyant to be able to see how FDA will escalate the regulatory pain.

Crafting a Response

The next steps taken by the CJO is to ensure a response is drafted and returned to the Agency within 15-days, not 15-weeks, 15-months, or 15-years. From FDA's perspective, a prompt and well-positioned response equates to an organization taking the Form 483 seriously. Dr. D recommends loading all 483 observations into the Corrective and Preventive Action (CAPA) system, regardless of how innocuous the observations might be. This way progress toward correcting each of the observations can be tracked individually. Additionally, it makes the review of actions pursued easier to review by the agency. Keeping it easy for FDA to understand is a good thing.

Furthermore, the response to the Form 483 should contain sufficient granularity so the agency understands the steps being pursued to correct the non-compliances. For example, in responding to the Form 483, the doctor recommends the following

information should be considered in the response:

- A restatement of the Form 483 Observation(s);

- A well-articulated corrective action plan (ensure past, current, and future states influenced by the observation are assessed);

- Reference to the CAPA number opened;

- Identification of root cause;

- Impact to product that has been shipped to customers;

- Impact to product currently being manufactured;

- Potential impact to future products;

- Impact to the quality management system;

- The targeted date for completion; and

- Other information deemed relevant to addressing the Form 483.

Finally, do not forget to add a cover letter to the response. Remember, a thorough

and well-thought out response to a Form 483 is an organization's best preemptive defense

in preventing the issuance of a warning letter. One final thought, make sure all of the

corrections are implemented and effective. Why? Because during the agency's next

friendly visit to your facility, they will revisit previous observations and verify they are

closed.

Takeaways

For this chapter, Dr. D will leave the readers with just one takeaway. It's okay to

disagree with a Form 483 observation; however, it is up to the offending organization to

draft a salient response that delineates the points of disagreement. If an organization

disagrees, it is incumbent upon the organization to provide supporting evidence as to why

they believe the observation has been incorrectly made. The FDA's expectation is that these types of disputes can be resolved as part of the inspection debrief; however, that is not always the case.

One final thought: never ever, ever, ever, ever inform the agency that the reason your organization cannot achieve compliance is because of resources constraints. As Dr. D has stated on multiple occasions, "Compliance to regulations is just part of the price of admission to play in the medical device industry." If an organization does not have or will not invest in adequate resources, they are playing in the wrong sandbox, consider making pet rocks as an alternative.

"It's okay to disagree with a Form 483 observation."

You Got a Warning Letter from FDA, Now What?

You Got a Warning Letter from FDA, Now What?

So your organization has received a warning letter from the FDA – now what? From the FDA's perspective, you either failed to respond promptly and completely to the Form 483 observations; or the agency just decided that your organization's QMS is irrevocably broken. For starters, the agency has quickly upped the ante in regards to taking the next steps in ensuring your organization clearly understands that a continued state of non-compliance is not acceptable. In short, the FDA issues warning letters when; (a) Form 483 responses are seriously deficient; (b) an organization has failed to respond to a Form 483, (c) the violations of the Act are so egregious, the FDA has decided to move rapidly to warning letter or (d) all of the above. In fact, the warning letter signifies the beginning of some serious regulatory whoop-ass being unleashed by the agency. Dr. D likes to call this FDA Purgatory. Once an organization migrates to under the umbrella of an FDA warning letter, business as usual comes to an abrupt end. The agency is no longer obliged to review and approve new product submissions. Can you say no PMA approvals? Additionally, letters needed by foreign governments for product exportation, a.k.a., FDA Export Certificates are no longer reviewed, approved, and signed. For medical device manufacturers these certificates are formally known as: (a) Certificate to Foreign Government; and (b) Certificate of Exportability. The impact to an organization's bottom line can be severe, as these certificates begin to expire. The amount of time spent in warning-letter land is entirely up to the organization and the number of objectionable conditions noted in the warning letter. If the responses formulated and sent to the agency lack depth and detail, and the FDA believes the responses are inadequate or ineffective, the time spent in the proverbial "land of lost opportunities" can be years. Dr. D strongly recommends the pulling out of all stops so organizations can quickly extricate themselves from FDA Purgatory. One thing your chief financial officer (CFO) will find out quickly is the healthy "*remuneration*" (look-it-up) paid to specialists capable of assisting in the cleanup of the warning letter mess. Folks - correcting a warning letter is never going to be cheap; and Dr. D says you can take that to the bank.

What is a Warning Letter?

Just because an organization is a Form 483 recipient, at the close of an inspection, does not necessarily translate into a warning letter. Upon conclusion of an inspection, the FDA investigator is tasked with writing the Establishment Inspection Report (EIR). The completed EIR will be reviewed at the local district office; and if the reviewer believes the content and evidence depicted in the EIR points to serious deficiencies in an establishment's quality system, then a warning letter will be issued. Additionally, as of April of 2009, the agency has adopted a policy of automatically issuing warning letters to establishments failing to respond to a Form 483 within the allotted 15-days. Ouch! There will be no susurrus (look-it-up) opening phrases in the initial paragraph of the FDA's warning letter. In fact, the warning letter's opening paragraph typically commences with, "*During an inspection of your firm*" and ends with "*Please notify this office in writing within fifteen (15) working days from the date you receive this letter of the specific steps you have taken to correct the noted violations, including an explanation of how you plan to prevent these violations, or similar violations, from occurring again. Include documentation of the corrective action you have taken.*"

According to the FDA, the issuance of a warning letter is one of the tools in their FDA enforcement bag. The purpose of the warning letter is to attempt to extract a voluntary correction of objectionable conditions by the agency. Remember, the issuance of a warning letter is not the final regulatory action available to the agency. In fact, Dr. D's position is the warning letter is the proverbial warning shot. As the doctor stated in the opening paragraph, the warning letter results in a significant interruptions in the day-to-day activities of the recipients.

What Happens Next?

The good news is that the US Marshalls have not shown up at your establishment's doorstep to chain and padlock the doors. More good news - a warning letter, although painful, is a recoverable event and can make an organization stronger. How does the saying go, "What doesn't kill you makes you stronger!" Dr. D strongly recommends that if the organization does not have the expertise to respond to the warning letter or does not retain legal counsel that understands the entire process, this expertise be acquired immediately. One thing an organization must remember is that the warning letter is not a simple overnight fix. Warning letters typically result in a protracted period where corrections to the objectionable conditions are achieved. This is not rocket science folks, the more observations depicted in the warning letter, the longer the stay in FDA Purgatory.

Responding to a Warning Letter

Responding to a warning letter is similar to that of a Form 483. Upon receipt of the warning letter, an organization has 15-working days to respond to the FDA. Additionally, the doctor strongly recommends that legal counsel review all correspondence with the agency. Once again, the recipient of the warning letter should draft a cover letter with all correspondences back to the agency. There will be several during the life of the warning letter so meticulous records of each submission should be kept. For example, in responding to the warning letter, the doctor recommends the following information should be considered in the response:

1. A restatement of the Form 483 Observation;

2. The proposed corrective action or plan (ensure past, current, and future states influenced by the observation are assessed);

3. Reference to the specific CAPA number;

4. Ensure root cause is determined and addressed;

5. Don't forget about the verification of effectiveness for all CAPAs pursued;

6. Potential impact to product;

7. Potential impact to the quality system; and

8. The targeted date for completion.

Warning Letter Watch outs – What Not to Do

Dr. D has a few watch outs he will share with the readers.

1. Never, never, never, never, complain the FDA has singled out your company and is intentionally picking on you. The argument will never fly.

2. Never fail to respond back to the agency, within the 15-days allotted or fail to meet committed dates made by your organization as part of the correction activities.

3. Remember, the agency will verify objectionable conditions have been closed prior to lifting the warning letter, so ensure all correction activities are closed prior to scheduling a follow-up visit by the agency.

4. Always provide the agency with sufficient detail and supporting documentation that reflects the actions pursued in support of the corrections.

5. If the corrections are going to take a significant amount of time, give the FDA reasonable timetable for correcting all of the objectionable conditions. Ensure that status updates are routinely provided to the agency.

6. Never downplay or minimize the seriousness of the observation. Remember, the FDA would not have issued the warning letter if they did not believe the enforcement action was warranted.

Takeaways

Yes, warning letters are life-changing events for device manufacturers; however, they are recoverable. Dr. D always recommends seeking legal counsel and industry experts involved when responding to a warning letter, reviewing subsequent correspondences to the agency, and the actual steps pursued in correction the objectionable conditions. Always remember, the FDA is not picking on you but they have a responsibility to protect public health. It is the agency's position that the objectionable conditions delineated within each waning letter could have an adverse effect on public health.

"Dr. D always recommends seeking legal counsel and industry experts involved when responding to a warning letter."

CAPA is Not Rocket Science

CAPA is not Rocket Science

The doctor is always amazed when he examines a CAPA system in which the owners swear up and down that their super-charged system is capable of "*obviating*" (look-it-up) all of their organizational woes. Sorry folks, but injecting the CAPA programs with steroids isn't the answer. In fact, the more complex the CAPA system, the more opportunities for Dr. D's good friend, Mr. Murphy to raise his head and unleash organizational mayhem. Please keep in mind, the FDA, Health Canada, MHLW, the Competent Authorities in Europe, etc., want a system that actually works. That being said, Dr. D's opinion is that it is best to keep the system simple. Simple CAPA system, good! Complex CAPA system on steroids, bad!

The doctor recommends pursuing Dr. D's 7-Step Model encompassing: (a) problem definition and scope; (b) initial investigation; (c) root-cause analysis; (d) proposed solution; (e) verification, validation, and implementation, (f) verification of effectiveness, and (g) documenting and sharing CAPA information. Remember to keep in mind the potential impact to product safety and efficacy, regulatory compliance, and overall quality system effectiveness, resulting from CAPA-driven changes to product, processes, and procedures.

Recent Warning Letter

The doctor has taken the liberty of extracting an excerpt from a March 5, 2013 warning letter, issued by our good friends from the agency.

Failure to establish and maintain procedures for implementing corrective and preventive action, as required by 21 CFR 820.100(a). For example, the corrective and preventive action procedure titled, "Improvement," Chapter 7 of PP8 Quality Management System procedure Rev. 0.9, has the following incomplete or missing requirements:

a) missing and incomplete requirements in Section 7.1, "Scope:" addressing the analysis of sources of quality data to identify existing and potential causes of nonconforming product, or other quality problems, and does not identify all sources of potential causes of nonconforming product or other quality data sources in the procedure;

b) no requirements for verifying or validating corrective or preventive actions prior to implementation, to ensure the actions do not adversely affect the devices;

c) missing requirement for assurance that all required activities are to be documented; and

d) no requirements for investigating the cause of nonconformities relating to processes, products, and the quality system.

Review of (b)(4) Corrective Action record, CAPA No. (b)(4), related to a U.S. marketed device, the Lumix 3 Ultra/Plus, did not reveal any of the required information as described above.

Problem Definition & Scope Phase

In this initial phase, the CAPA owner is doing nothing more than providing some initial framework for the CAPA. Basically, the CAPA form is opened and critical information surrounding the non-conformance is collected. Depending on the nature of the problem, initial target dates may be identified. However, moving into the initial investigational phase should occur as quickly as possible.

Initial Investigation Phase

The initial investigation phase associated with CAPA is pretty cut and dry. The QSR requires device manufacturers to investigate the cause of **ALL** product issues (nonconformities), process issues, and quality system issues. Remember, device manufacturers are not free to pick and choose the problems they want to resolve. Device manufacturers need to fix all nonconformities that have been identified. Additionally, device manufacturers need to exhibit a sense of urgency in executing investigations. One year, or even longer, is just too damned long to complete an initial investigation.

Furthermore, if the agency determines the approach to CAPA investigations is

unsatisfactory, the device manufacturer can expect to receive a Form 483, during their

next friendly FDA inspection.

Root-Cause Analysis Phase

So what are regulators looking for in regards to root-cause analysis? In short,

regulators want device manufacturers to continually monitor all aspect of their operation

and use the results, if warranted, as quality inputs into the CAPA system. For example,

unfavorable trends in yields discovered on the manufacturing floor, a nonconformance

discovered during an internal quality audit, returned product, and product complaints are

a few examples of quality inputs requiring input into the CAPA system. The QSR

specifically adds a callout for "other sources of data" and "other quality problems." These

catchall phrases equate to considering all potential and actual quality problems for

inclusion into the CAPA system or an "all-encompassing approach." Remember two of

the salient purposes of CAPA are; (a) to prevent problems from occurring, and (b)

prevention of problem recurrence once a problem has occurred.

However, please do not forget, root-cause is root-cause. What? Seriously folks,

there is no value in providing a less than robust root-cause analysis. Feel free to employ

the tools the QA gods, such as Dr. Deming gave to us all. So why is root cause so darned

important? If you have to ask then you are in the wrong business. If root cause does not

correctly identify the underlying problem, the proposed solution is probably not going to

work. Simply stated; "A crappy investigation results in the development of a crappy

solution."

Proposed Solution Phase

The expectation of regulators is that once a CAPA investigation is complete and root-cause identified, the appropriate actions needing to correct nonconformities should be identified. The doctor would like to warn the readers against using too many concessions such as "no-further action is required due to an isolated incident" or an oldie but a goody "no obvious trend." Device manufacturers that frequently invoke concessions are typically awarded with Form 483s observations questioning the effectiveness of their CAPA system. That said, once the appropriate actions have been identified, Dr. D strongly recommends moving into the validation, verification, and implementation of the proposed solutions.

Validation, Verification, and Implementation Phase

Although device manufacturers are typically pretty confident when they move into their implementing solution phase, they must first determine if the proposed action is going to have a negative impact on product safety and efficacy of finished devices. Dr. D is pretty positive, well maybe somewhat positive; device manufacturers do a good job performing in-depth root-cause analysis, while identifying potential corrections to problems. However, regulators want device manufacturers to be absolutely sure there is no potential negative impact to finished devices, prior to implementing changes.

Moving to implementation, device manufacturers need to ensure all changes are documented. Dr. D's not so secret approach is to employ the change request process that feeds the document control system. All changes need to be reviewed and approved. Additionally, changes made to product need to be captured within the Design History File (DHF). Furthermore, ensure FMEAs are reassessed for potential changes in levels of risk

46

and/or occurrences. Finally, make sure your organization's regulatory affairs group is involved with reviewing all product changes. Why? Product changes, depending on device class and regulatory authority involved, may require pre-approval prior to releasing the product into the market place, e.g., PMA supplement for Class III product in the US.

Verification of Effectiveness (VOE) Phase

Now Dr. D is going to climb out on a limb here and assume the readers are performing VOE phase. If not, what are you waiting for? If the CAPA resulted in a minor change to a procedure or a dimensional change to a mechanical drawing, then VOE can occur ASAP. However, if the change driven by CAPA was to correct a systemic issue, then 90-days is a realistic approach for returning to the proverbial "scene of the crime" and verifying that actions taken were effective and suitable for the risk. Over the years, the doctor has examined far-too-many CAPA systems were the VOE step is missing from the process.

Documenting and Sharing CAPA Information Phase

Information is and always will be a powerful tool. It should be incumbent upon all device manufacturers to ensure information associated with quality problems, nonconforming product, and potential quality issues be disseminated amongst the proverbial ranks. Successful dissemination of information, i.e., Kaizen circles, etc., will result in the prevention of problem recurrence. For example, if there have been MDRs or vigilance reports opened that identify tip separation from a catheter, and the failure investigation determines the root-cause is process related, the operators on the manufacturing floor need to be made aware of the process problem. Otherwise, "history will repeat itself."

Takeaways

I think the most important takeaway, for this chapter, is to use the CAPA system to fix all of your quality problems. A strong CAPA system will allow organizations to track quality problems to closure. Additionally, when problems are identified or potential problems noted, device manufacturers need to act quickly. If you ever want to see Dr. D angry, one way to do it quickly is to place a problem or other nonconformance into the CAPA system; and then take over a year to resolve an issue that should have been corrected in a few days or worst case a couple of weeks. In fact, that type of performance will quickly grab the attention of regulators as well. Remember CAPA is not rocket science. You identify problems and you fix problems.

The expectation of regulators is that once a CAPA investigation is complete and root-cause identified, the appropriate actions needing to correct nonconformities should be identified.

Not all Suppliers Need Audits

Not all Suppliers Need Audits

Dr. D has some very good news for the readers. Medical device manufacturers are not required to audit their suppliers. But hey, if you do not believe the doctor, Dr. D has taken the time to cut-and-paste the requirement from §820.50 (Purchasing Controls). Remember it is not by some "*perforce*" (look-it-up) bias that the doctor choses to write, Dr. D writes to teach and clarify.

Each manufacturer shall establish and maintain procedures to ensure that all purchased or otherwise received product and services conform to specified requirements.

> *(a) Evaluation of suppliers, contractors, and consultants. Each manufacturer shall establish and maintain the requirements, including quality requirements, that must be met by suppliers, contractors, and consultants. Each manufacturer shall:*
>
> *(1) Evaluate and select potential suppliers, contractors, and consultants on the basis of their ability to meet specified requirements, including quality requirements. The evaluation shall be documented.*
>
> *(2) Define the type and extent of control to be exercised over the product, services, suppliers, contractors, and consultants, based on the evaluation results.*
>
> *(3) Establish and maintain records of acceptable suppliers, contractors, and consultants.*
>
> *(b) Purchasing data. Each manufacturer shall establish and maintain data that clearly describe or reference the specified requirements, including quality requirements, for purchased or otherwise received product and services. Purchasing documents shall include, where possible, an agreement that the suppliers, contractors, and consultants agree to notify the manufacturer of changes in the product or service so that manufacturers may determine whether the changes may affect the quality of a finished device. Purchasing data shall be approved in accordance with 820.40.*

Now, that you have taken the time to read it, please point out to the doctor where it mentions that an audit of suppliers are mandatory. How about ISO 13485:2003? Will you find the need to audit suppliers scripted there? Once again, the good doctor has taken the opportunity to cut-and-paste Clause 7.4.1 of ISO 13485:2003 (Purchasing Process).

- *The organization shall establish documented procedures to ensure that purchased   product conforms to specified purchase requirements.*

- *The type and extent of control applied to the supplier and the purchased product shall be dependent upon the effect of the purchased product on subsequent product realization or the final product.*

- *The organization shall evaluate and select suppliers based on their ability to supply product in accordance with the organization's requirements. Criteria for selection, evaluation and re-evaluation shall be established. Records of the results of evaluations and any necessary actions arising from the evaluation shall be maintained (see 4.2.4).*

Can you point out where supplier audits are mandated by clause 7.4.1? Of course you can't, because the requirement does not exist. So why bother auditing suppliers? The salient requirement is to evaluate supplier and select premised on requirements. How a device manufacturers does this is entirely up to them. In this chapter, the doctor is going to explain why some audits are necessary and most are not. Enjoy.

Let's Start with Understanding Risk

You would not buy a car without test driving it first, so why would a device manufacturer attempt to purchase product from a new supplier without visiting and kicking the proverbial tires? For medical device manufacturers, it is incumbent upon the organization to investigate the capabilities of potential suppliers prior to the commencement of any procurement activities. I strongly recommend starting with the moderately famous and extremely useful D & B, and no, I am not a paid spokesperson for this service. The Dunn & Bradstreet report provides a condensed business synopsis on potential suppliers and can save an organization from much grief and pain if potential suppliers have cash flow issues, pending litigation, or other significant problems that can influence their business both short and long term. Remember; if a potential supplier is experiencing business problems, those problems will quickly become the problem of your organization, if the decision is made to proceed with the relationship. Now I am not implying the D & B should be the all-encompassing selection tool; however, it should carry some weight in regards to the selection process.

The second important factor relating to risk is the potential failure of a procured component and the influence a failed component could have on the finished medical device. I strongly recommend, early in the design and development process, linking the component failure risk back to the design and preferably to the design Failure Mode and Effects Analysis (dFMEA). Additionally, best-in-class industry practices drive the alignment of suppliers into categories premised on risk and organizational need (reference Table 1.0). For example, when selecting a supplier for providing a disposable manufacturing aide such as finger cots, the selection and evaluation process will differ dramatically from that of a contract manufacturer.

Requirements Driven Supplier Evaluation Process

You would not buy a house without sharing with your real-estate agent some basic requirements as to what your needs are, i.e., size, rooms, location, etc. Well, guess what? The supplier selection process cannot commence until basic requirements and needs are defined by your organization. For all of you engineers used to working from a napkin drawing, once your ideas are captured and formulated, a formal document really needs to be created, e.g., component specification. Additionally, when defining these requirements the approach pursued must be cross-functional. Yes, engineers are driving the train because they are tasked with owning the design and development. However, quality, regulatory, manufacturing, procurement, materials, supply chain, marketing, etc. are key stakeholders; and should provide input into the selection process. Furthermore, if a candidate supplier possesses a quality system certified by a recognized registrar or notified body, the premise of the initial supplier visit can be focused on process and overall business capabilities. Finally, because developing suppliers and qualifying material is expensive, never let one functional group be the sole stakeholder in the selection process. The final decision to approve and add a supplier to your organization's Approved Vendor's List (AVL) must be a collaborative one.

Different Approaches to Supplier Audits

Yes, believe it or not there are different types of supplier audits. Remember, there is no one-shoe-fits-all approach. Let's face it there are some suppliers you are going to need to visit. High-risk suppliers (quality, regulatory, or business-risk related), critical component suppliers, sterilization facilities, and contract manufacturers should be on the list for an on-site audit. Yes, trust is important; however, there is too much risk at stake by not visiting these suppliers. In fact, Dr. D recommends an annual visit for suppliers considered high-risk.

The doctor also recommends developing a core set of quality/compliance related questions that can be used for all audits. These questions should align with ISO 13485 or 21 CFR, Part 820, as applicable. The balance of questions for an on-site audit should be commodity specific. For example, if the audit is being performed at EO sterilization facility, then the process-related questions should be ISO 11135-1 centric. If the audit is of a testing laboratory or a metrology supplier, the process-related questions should be ISO/IEC 17025 centric.

So what are the different types of supplier audits that can be used to establish evidence that the approach to supplier selection and supplier management is effective? The doctor has identified four types of assessments that are defendable during and audit or inspection, providing the supporting SOP adequately defines the process:

1. On-site supplier audit (full QMS & process assessment);

2. On-site focused audit (targeting a specific problem or process);

3. Mail-in audit (basic supplier questionnaire used to compile QMS and basic business information); and

4. Telephone (desk-top) audit (Request for a copy of the ISO certificate(s); quality manual; and list of SOPs supporting the QMS).

The next logical question needing to be asked is; "What is the frequency of supplier re-evaluations?" The doctor's answer is, "It depends." The doctor recommends auditing critical suppliers at least once a year. However, just like initial supplier audits, re-evaluation audits need to be premised on risk (business, quality, and regulatory). Table 1 reflects the categorization of suppliers premised on risk.

Table 1.0 – Supplier Categorization Premised on Risk

Category & Assessment	Applicability	Re-Audit Frequency
Category 1 *Annual On-Site Assessment Mandatory – Due to Risk*	• Contract Manufacturers, Sterilization Facility	Annually
Category 2 *On-Site Assessment Mandatory (Premised on Schedule & Risk)*	• Components Identified as Critical Premised on the Device FMEA • Laboratory Services Providers • Analytical Test Labs • Calibration/Metrology Provider • Notified Bodies	Two-Years
Category 3 *On-Site Assessment is optional (Premised on Risk) / Mail-In Survey Required*	• Non-Critical Custom Material, Process, and/or Component • Offsite Record Storage • Environmental Services Provider	Three-Years

Category & Assessment	Applicability	Re-Audit Frequency
Category 4 *Mail-In Survey is optional (providing certifications are current)* Current ISO 9001 or ISO 13485 Certificates; Lead Auditor Certificate; Resume, etc., are acceptable in lieu of survey.	• Standard Catalog Component Manufacturers • Low-Risk Components • Distributors of Catalog Components • Consultants • Facility Services, i.e., Janitorial Services, Pest Control, etc.	When Certificates Expire
Category 5 No Requirement for Quality System Assessments – Purchase Order Only	• Transportation Services (UPS, USPS, etc.) • Disposable Supplies (wipes, finger cots, etc.)	N/A

Takeaways

I think the most important takeaway, from this chapter is the understanding that supplier audits are important tools; however, regulations and standards give device manufacturers much flexibility when implementing a supplier audit program that is effective for their organization. Should suppliers by audited? Absolutely; however, the doctor recommends pursuing a common-sense approach when scripting an audit program. If you need help, fell free to contact Dr. D at chris.devine@devineguidanceinternational.com. Creating a supplier audit program or assisting is the execution of supplier audits is one of the core competencies of Devine Guidance.

You would not buy a car without test driving it first, so why would a device manufacturer attempt to purchase product from a new supplier without visiting and kicking the proverbial tires?

SCARs – Dr. D Loves the Acronym

SCARs – Dr. D Loves the Acronym

The doctor would like start this chapter's Guidance with a couple of questions. Can the readers point to Dr. D where the use of a Supplier Corrective Action Request (SCAR) is required within 21 CFR, Part 820 (the FDA's Quality System Regulation)? How about within ISO 13485:2003? The doctor will provide the answers for the readers just in case some of you might have to look. The answer is "NO" to both questions; and "NO" Dr. D is not being "*persnickety*" (look-it-up). Getting back to SCAR, device manufacturers really do need a vehicle for communicating and documenting supplier problems. Yes, the doctor said documenting. Why? Because if an action is not documented in writing, in the eyes of FDA (not one of the doctors favorite acronyms), the action never occurred; kind of like Bill Clinton smoking a joint but never inhaling. That being said, Dr. D hopes you enjoy this chapter's guidance.

The doctor is just full of questions so here goes another one. Do all supplier non-conformances require a SCAR? The answer is a resounding 'NO!" For example, if a supplier sends a Certificate of Conformance (C of C) containing a typographical error or an incorrect quantity, it is acceptable to call the supplier and ask that this issue be remedied ASAP (another great acronym). This is called effective communication. However, if the supplier makes the same error again, the correct path would be to SCAR (God the doctor loves this acronym) the supplier. Let's talk about the SCAR process. Dr. D believes in having two categories of SCARs: (a) Information Only – no response required; and (b) Response Required. The doctor used to have a third category "Terminate Supplier with Extreme Prejudice." However, after several months there were no suppliers remaining on the Approved Suppliers List (ASL – another good acronym); just kidding about the category folks. Seriously, if the problem is really benign, and more than a phone call is required, Dr. D recommends issuing an "Information Only Scar." If the problem is more severe such as component dimensional issues, test failures, process steps missing (e.g., missing anodize), etc. then a "Response Required" SCAR is probably the correct path to pursue.

The next question coming from the inquisitive Dr. D is: "What is the appropriate time period for a supplier to respond to a SCAR?" The answer is it depends and not the adult diaper version. Typically, 30-days has always been an acceptable standard. However, if the supplier issue has resulted in Medical Device Reports (MDR's – another valuable acronym) or even worse a product **RECALL**, Dr. D's favorite six-letter word, then 5-working days is not an unreasonable request. The doctor's best advice is to premise the required response time on the appropriate level of risk.

The next logical question pertains to evaluating a suppliers SCAR response. How should device manufacturers evaluate a suppliers SCAR response? For starters, if a supplier has failed to respond, the problem needs to be quickly elevated to the supplier's management. If a supplier refuses to respond, then find a new supplier. There are too many good suppliers in this world to suffer through having a non-responsive or arrogant one. When evaluating a SCAR response the doctor looks for three things.

- What action has the supplier taken in regards to immediate containment?
- What action has the supplier taken rectify the problem and ensure acceptable product is manufactured and shipped?
- What action has the supplier taken to prevent future recurrences?

If the supplier has provided a reasonable response it all boils down to verification of effectiveness (VOE – another acronym for the readers). If the supplier issue is not an Earth-shattering problem, then accepting the suppliers VOE should suffice. Since Dr. D strongly believes in phrase made famous by Deming; "In God we trust all others bring data," it is strongly recommended that a review of all SCAR VOEs be assessed during supplier audits. On another note, if a supplier is racking up SCARs, regardless of their responsiveness, it just might be time to qualify a new supplier. Finally, SCAR information should be included in supplier report cards.

Takeaways

For this chapter, the doctor will leave the readers with a few pearls of wisdom. It is imperative that medical device manufacturers have a tool for communicating supplier issues back to their suppliers. Yes, a phone call is probably ok for a minor issue; however, it is always better to have documentation. Why? You just don't know when the Agency might show up on your doorstep for a cup of coffee and an inspection. The issuance of an "Information Only" versus a "Response Required" SCAR is really driven by risk. If a response is required from the supplier, make sure the supplier actually responds and the response is adequate.

"The doctor used to have a third category of SCAR; "Terminate Supplier with Extreme Prejudice!"

Nonconforming Product

Nonconforming Product

In a perfect world, money grows on trees, good bourbon flows freely from the garden hose, Cuban cigars are legal to smoke, and the San Jose Sharks win Lord Stanley's Cup. Unfortunately, Mr. Murphy is alive and well in the medical device industry, and as a result it is inevitable that device manufacturers will have to handle non-conforming product. If a device manufacturer has *"exiguous" (look-it-up)* policies and procedures for handling nonconforming product, then it will never be a question as to if FDA will pay a visit but when the FDA will pay a visit to the device manufacturer's facility

Nonconforming Product

The effective handling of nonconforming product is essential for all device manufacturers. Identifying, quarantining, investigating, and correcting, are salient steps that need to be completed when dealing with nonconforming product. Trust Dr. D when I say, "the mishandling of nonconforming product can be costly, may result in product withdraws (RECALLS), and invite a surprise visit from the FDA." Identification is only a small piece to solving the handling of nonconforming product puzzle. The best guidance Dr. D can offer to the readers is to invest in developing an effective process for managing nonconforming product. The process should include:

- Robust procedures;

- A well-designed form, e.g., Non-conforming Material Report (NCMR);

- A link to CAPA;

- A clearly-defined process for disposition;

- The creation of nonconforming-product tags;

- A segregated storage area (restricted-access quarantine location);

- Instructions for rework;

- Supplier notification or supplier corrective action request (SCAR), if warranted;

- A policy for returning nonconforming product to the supplier; and

- A Material Review Board (MRB) process.

Control of Nonconforming Product

The need for an investigation, root-cause analysis, and the notification (when applicable) of the appropriate organizations (internal and external) are required when nonconforming product is identified. If the nonconformance is determined to be external, a.k.a., supplier generated, a SCAR should be issued to prevent a recurrence of the nonconformance. Additionally, ensure all SCAR activity is closed with a verification of effectiveness step; otherwise, history will repeat itself, just ask Mr. Murphy. Furthermore, all of these activities shall be documented. Why – "because documented evidence of compliance is your best defense during a friendly visit from the agency."

Nonconformity Review and Disposition

For starters, you should never have manufacturing be the sole authority for providing disposition of nonconforming product. As a minimum, the doctor recommends including, (a) manufacturing, (b) purchasing, (c) quality, (d) supply chain, (e) R & D, (f) manufacturing engineering; (g) quality engineering and (h) the janitor (just kidding on the janitor). Extended reviewers, employed as necessary, can be (a) clinical / medical sciences, (b) marketing, (c) sales, and (d) the cafeteria staff "sorry, just kidding again on the cafeteria staff." Additionally, all dispositions require more than just names; signatures and dates are also needed. Furthermore, Dr. D **STRONGLY RECOMMENDS** that use-as-is (UAI) never is used for Class III devices. A UAI disposition implies product does not meet specification and a conveyance is required to accept the product. In short, the nonconforming product now meets a different specification, probably wider. This equates to a design change. Now you can argue with the doctor until the cows come home, but you will never win this argument. Why? Because design changes made to Class III products require a PMA supplement (as a minimum) and subsequent review and approval by the agency. The doctor's recommendation will always be to rework nonconforming product to print, scrap and remanufacture, or return the nonconforming product to the supplier (with a nasty gram of course). The regulatory risk is just too high. Finally, document the results. Why? Broken-record time; "because documented evidence of compliance is your best defense during a friendly visit from the agency."

Rework

Rework of nonconforming product is an area where Dr. D sees device manufacturers often getting themselves into trouble. You already know Dr. D's position on UAI. That being said, rework, which means reworking nonconforming product to established and approved specifications, is a viable option. As part of the rework process, the agency's expectation is that the product be retested and/or reevaluated to ensure compliance to the product's approved specification is achieved. If the current product specification is not approved or has been changed and not approved, your organization has other issues. These issues will quickly be exacerbated when the agency stops by for a cup of coffee and an inspection.

Reworked product needs to be assessed for potential long-term impact to product performance, a.k.a., product safety and efficacy. What? For example, let say a finished-device lot has been sterilized employing Ethylene Oxide (EO). While attempting to load the finished devices onto a truck for shipment to distribution a forklift driver (true story) has managed to attack a pallet containing the product with the forks of the forklift. As part of the disposition, it has been determined the product will be inspected, repackaged, submitted to EO sterilization for a second time, and released for distribution. If the finished devices were only validated for one sterilization cycle (1X), you now have a problem. That is why all aspects of the rework need to be evaluated. Furthermore, all rework activities shall be documented and placed into the Device History Record (DHR).

Finally, Dr. D recommends the DHR be maintained in a pristine condition as accuracy counts. Trust me, the FDA will look at your DHRs and use the review as one of the stepping-off point for their inspection, along with CAPA. Remember, the DHR contains the entire manufacturing history for each device or lot of finished devices. Finally, a complete and accurate DHR is extremely important; "because documented evidence of compliance is your best defense during a friendly visit from the agency."

Takeaways

Dr. D cannot place enough emphasis on not taking shortcuts when it comes to the handling of nonconforming product. Managing nonconforming product effectively begins with the creation of a robust written procedure. Other important aspects associated with the control of nonconforming product are: (a) clear identification of all nonconforming product; (b) restricted-access quarantine locations; (c) a well-defined disposition policy; (d) MRB meetings; (e) the use of clearly-defined rework instructions; and (f) a link to the device manufacturer's CAPA system (internal and supplier).

*"Managing nonconforming product
effectively begins with the creation of
a robust written procedure!"*

Detention

Detention

For this chapter, Dr. D will briefly discuss detention. Now as a youngster, the doctor was well-versed in the virtues of detention as Dr. D spent hours-upon-hours thinking about the need to correct one's behavior. Sorry Mr. Principal, I did not think putting some Ex-lax in my teacher's coffee was a big deal. The doctor was only trying to prove a point in biology class. Seriously folks the concept of detention, employed by FDA, is not unlike the pain associated with the after school detention of this doctor's wayward youth. The principal places you in a room and you cannot leave. However, the FDA's pain will hit a device manufacturer squarely in the pocket. In searching through the FDA's warning letter database for this chapter's guidance, the doctor came upon a recent letter issued to Lucky Board Manufacturing. Unfortunately, Lucky Board Manufacturing just may be contemplating a name change to "Unlucky" Board Manufacturing. You see, Lucky has been manufacturing and selling surgical masks without one minor little detail; they lack pre-market approval as required by the Act. Now granted, surgical masks can be categorized as a *"fungible"* (look-it-up) commodity; however, approval/clearance is still required to enter these devices into commerce in the United States. Just maybe, someone at Lucky might want to consider reading 21 CFR, Part 807.

FDA Warning Letter Issued on June 20, 2013

Given the serious nature of the violations of the Act, surgical masks manufactured by your firm are subject to refusal of admission under section 801(a) of the Act, 21 U.S.C. § 381(a), in that they appear to be adulterated. As a result, FDA may take steps to refuse these products, known as "detention without physical examination," until these violations are corrected. In order to remove the devices from detention, your firm should provide a written response to this Warning Letter as described below and correct the violations described in this letter. We will notify you if your firm's response appears to be adequate, and we may need to re-inspect your firm's facility to verify that the appropriate corrections and/or corrective actions have been made.

Detention

For this chapter, the doctor will be brief. The FDA retains the right to seize and place into detention adulterated product, including the refusal to admit violative products into the United States. Our good friends at Lucky will need to satisfy all of the concerns noted in the warning letter, including the filing of a pre-market application for their device, to once again fall within the good graces of the agency. Please keep in mind, the process of correcting a warning letter is not cheap. Not only are the dollars or in this case the Yuan, going to quickly add up, but the lost revenue from sales in the United States is going to severely impinge upon this organization's bottom line. Additionally, the warning letter mitigation process is time consuming. For all of you wannabe CFO's out there, time equates to money. Duh, real rocket science from Dr. D. Seriously, warning letters are not resolved in a few days, a few weeks, or even a few months. Depending on the organization's response and commitment, a warning letter could take a year or even longer to correct. I would think detention or the threat of detention would be sufficient to correct the behavior of noncompliance. Heck it worked for the doctor as a high school student.

Takeaways

For this chapter's guidance, Dr. D will leave the readers with one takeaway. The FDA wields an incredible amount of power when it comes to enforcing compliance to the Act. Detention is just one of the tools in the FDA's tool chest. As a device industry professional, the doctor cannot fathom how a device manufacturer fails to acknowledge the need to obtain clearance from the FDA for a device being introduced into commerce

in the United States, regardless of the country of origin. Folks, remember only devices

categorized as Class I exempt are "EXEMPT" from the pre-market approval process.

Duh, do you think!

"The FDA wields an incredible amount of power when it comes to enforcing compliance to the Act."

Product Seizures

Product Seizures

Product seizure is always an interesting topic to explore. The doctor finds the concept of seizure fascinating, especially when it results in the government performing the actual taking of violative medical devices. Thank God it doesn't happen too often. It is Dr. D's humble opinion that if a device manufacturer has had product seized due to compliance issues or egregious violations of the Act, then their quality and regulatory organizations must be run by "***addlepated***" (look-it-up) idiots. For this chapter's guidance the doctor will provide some insight into the concept of Product Seizure. Now granted, the seizure process is just a tiny bit more complex than having U.S. Marshalls kicking in the doors and backing up and loading the proverbial turnip truck. However, make no mistake seizure is one of the more powerful tools in the FDA's compliance tool chest. They have ways of making you comply. Enjoy.

FDA's Definition of Seizure

A seizure is a civil court action against a specific quantity of goods which enables FDA to remove these goods from commercial channels. After seizure, no one may tamper with the goods except by permission of the court. The court usually gives the owner or claimant of the seized merchandise approximately 30 days to decide a course of action. If they take no action, the court will recommend disposal of the goods. If the owner decides to contest the government's charges, the court will schedule the case for trial. A third option allows the owner of the goods to request permission of the court to bring the goods into compliance with the law. The owner of the goods is required to provide a bond (security deposit) to assure that they will perform the orders of the court, and the owner must pay for FDA supervision of any activities by the company to bring the goods into compliance.

Typical FDA Warning Letter Clause

Your firm should take prompt action to correct the violations addressed in this letter. Failure to promptly correct these violations may result in regulatory action being initiated by the FDA without further notice. These actions include, but are not limited to, *__seizure__, injunction, and civil money penalties. Also, federal agencies may be advised of the issuance of Warning Letters about devices so that they may take this information into account when considering the award of contracts.*

Product Seizures

Product seizure is a powerful enforcement tool, available to FDA, used to address compliance issues or quickly block medical devices that violate the Act or are deemed not to be safe and effective in their intended use. The good news is the FDA cannot just kick-in the doors. The agency needs a court order to proceed with the product seizure and eventual impounding of violative devices. Conversely, the government **does not** have to reimburse medical device manufacturers for the product seized. The bottom line is simple, just comply baby.

To give the readers a better idea of how frequently product seizures are employed by FDA, Table 1.0 contains a breakdown of product seizures. In most cases, the product seizures are warranted in protecting the health of the general public. However, in one highly-publicized case, industry experts believe the FDA may have over-reacted.

Year	Number of Product Seizures
2009	8
2010	10
2011	15
2012	8

Table 1.0 – FDA Product Seizures

An example of the potential over reaction of FDA's seizure process can be viewed in a highly-visible product seizure case from 2007. The FDA seized all implantable medical devices from a New Jersey-based medical device manufacturer in April of 2007. The FDA claimed the seizure was driven by the identification of significant deficiencies noted during a plant inspection. The FDA warned Shelhigh, Inc.

of the consequences associated with their failure to address violations noted during a previous inspection. Although there was a few minor compliance issues noted during the Shelhigh inspection, some device industry experts believe FDA's actions were not warranted. In fact, there was an underlying concern of the agency's ability to act with impunity. Eventually, Shelhigh and FDA agreed to an out-of-court settlement.

Takeaways

For this chapter's guidance, the doctor will leave the readers with just one takeaway. Common sense precludes the need for any relationship with FDA to sour to the point when a product seizure becomes eminent. The FDA is usually a reasonable agency to work with when a good-faith effort is being made to sustain quality and regulatory compliance. If observational deficiencies are noted during an inspection and a Form 483 is issued, address the darn deficiencies. Failure to do so will result in a Warning Letter and additional requests to respond to FDA will result in an eventual visit to the courts.

"Product seizure is a powerful enforcement tool, available to FDA!"

Can You Say Recall?

Recalls

Can you say Dr. D's favorite-ugly 6-letter word, RECALL? As the late Mr. Rogers would say, "I know you could." In a perfect world, there are no taxes, Cuban cigars are legal, good bourbon is always free, and the San Jose Sharks finally win Lord Stanley's Cup. Unfortunately, this world is far from perfect and the medical device industry even far less than perfect. Eventually, all medical device manufacturers will have to deal with at least one product recall. The more products being introduced into the US marketplace and the chances for a recall begin to increase significantly. One of the underlying reasons recalls occur is because good-ole Mr. Murphy is alive and well in the device industry. In fact, Mr. Murphy continues to actively breed. That being said, the FDA has very clear and concise policies pertaining to "removals and corrections" delineated within 21 CFR, Part 806. The doctor strongly suggests that for those readers not familiar with Part 806, there is no time like the present to start reading it. Part 806 can often be viewed by many as an "*inscrutable*" (look-it-up) piece of regulatory text than is often misconstrued. However, the FDA will use every tool at their disposal to force the removal of medical devices that are not safe and effective from the US market. Enjoy!

Recall

For those regulatory purists out there, Dr. D has a simple question for you. Do you know how many times the word RECALL is mentioned in Part 806? If you answered zero, the big goose egg, you would be correct. Although industry frequently employs the term recall, Part 806 provides definitions for four basic terms associated with getting bad devices or devices violative of the Act out of the US market: (a) correction; (b) market withdraw; (c) removal; and (d) stock recovery. Regardless of the term, the agency's message is loud and clear; "keep bad medical devices out of the American marketplace.

Part 806

Dr. D is not going to dive into Part 806 and give the readers a blow-by-blow take on the actual requirements. Since Part 806 is a relatively brief document, the doctor will allow the readers to scan Part 806 on their own time. However, Dr. D will provide some insight into the salient points associated with executing an effective recall.

For starters, you just might want to consider beginning with the scripting of a well-written procedure defining your organization's approach to recall management. The procedure should incorporate all of the little nuances associated with the FDA-mandated requirements delineated within Part 806. Make sure you focus on the customer notification process, the product recovery process, good-faith effort process, effectiveness checks, the reporting process to FDA, and the certified destruction process. If your company is in the infant stages of your organizational development, then the doctor strongly suggest investing in an ERP/MRP system that will allow for superb product traceability, including product shipments. Why? Because when Mr. Murphy comes knocking, it will just be a matter of time before the word RECALL will raise its ugly little head. Executing a successful recall will be driven by knowing where all of the suspect medical devices reside: (a) with a healthcare organization; (b) on a consignment shelf, (c) sitting on a shelf in a distribution center; (d) in transit; or (e) in the infamous trunk stock location, a.k.a., in the back of a sales rep's car or in the rep's garage.

Recall Classes

The FDA has identified three categories of recalls, each premised on risk to public health and safety. The recall class will drive the level of attention to detail and FDA involvement with the recall process.

Recall Classifications

These guidelines categorize all recalls into one of three classes, according to the level of hazard and risk involved:

> *"Class I:* ***Dangerous or defective products that predictably could cause serious health problems or death. Examples include: food found to contain botulinum toxin, food with undeclared allergens, a label mix-up on a lifesaving drug, or a defective artificial heart valve.***
>
> *Class II:* ***Products that might cause a temporary health problem, or pose only a slight threat of a serious nature. Example: a drug that is under-strength but that is not used to treat life-threatening situations.***
>
> *Class III:* ***Products that are unlikely to cause any adverse health reaction, but that violate FDA labeling or manufacturing laws. Examples include: a minor container defect and lack of English labeling in a retail food."***

The classification of a particular recall will define the boundaries for executing the recovery process. For the most part, product recalls are voluntary; however, the FDA giveth and the FDA taketh away. If a medical device poses an imminent threat to public health and safety, the agency can order a Class I recall. Even for a device-manufacturer sponsored recall, FDA notification is required. Through the concept of *"**First Alert"*** the FDA becomes aware of a product issue and the clock starts ticking.

Executing the Class I Recall

Right after the call is made to FDA for the initial consultation, the device manufacturer begins the arduous task of identifying where the medical devices requiring to be recalled are located within the United States. Written notification will be required.

In fact, ensure evidence of notification is collected, e.g., use FedEx, UPS or USPS to ship the recall packets and collect evidence of receipt. Just in case you are wondering, evidence of receipt equates to a signature acknowledging receipt of the recall package. In the eyes Dr. D and the FDA, the magic number is three, which equates to three attempts to collect product being recalled. Collecting the suspect devices will require significant vigilance and a recall manager with the persistence and tenacity of a pit bill, ruff, ruff! As product is returned and collected, it is imperative that the product be placed into a quarantine location and meticulous records associated with the recall maintained. Once the device manufacturer is in a position to accurately determine that no more devices are going to be returned, hopefully an effectiveness rate of greater than 90.0%, then FDA can be contacted and plans for the certified destruction of the devices executed. Once upon a time, in a distant land called California, Dr. D watched in amazement as a forklift was driven back and forth over a couple of hundred catheters in an effort to destroy them. Was it effective, heck yes; however, it was also quite messy. The doctor recommends contacting a firm specializing in the certified destruction of medical devices. Make sure the certificate of destruction is included in the recall documentation.

Dr. D strongly recommends pursuing the same rigor when executing a Class II or Class III device recall. Remember, the FDA will want to look at all of the documentation associated with a recall as part of one of their friendly visits, a.k.a., facility inspection. The agency is always interested in the effectiveness of a device manufacturer's recall efforts, regardless of the classification.

Takeaways

For this chapter's guidance, the doctor will leave the readers with two takeaways. One - It is inevitable a device manufacturer will eventually have to execute a product recall. The best policy is to always be prepared. In preparation, begin with scripting a procedure that fully embraces 21 CFR, Part 806. Two – It is imperative that FDA be kept in the loop for product recalls. Always, contact your local FDA office prior to commencing with a recall. The discussion with FDA will ensure that correct classification of recall is selected.

"The agency is always interested in the effectiveness of a device manufacturer's recall efforts, regardless of the classification!"

Failure to Define

Failure to Define

In FDA speak, the phrase *"failure to define"* is code for "your organization has screwed up and missed something!" Seriously folks complying with the FDA's Quality System Regulation (21 CFR, Part 820) does not entail rocket science. Repeat after Dr. D; "Rocket science no, common sense yes." The reason the doctor is writing about "failure to define" is that Dr. D came across an interesting warning letter. One of the Form 483 Observations noted in a warning letter date 03 July 2013 stated:

> *"Failure to define the type and extent of control to be exercised over suppliers, as required by 21 CFR 820.50(a)(2). Specifically, Your Purchasing Process and Supplier Evaluation Process Map (7.4.1) is ambiguous on how you will monitor your suppliers. Your process map lists the "input" for monitoring trends of performance as identifying performance parameters for suppliers. These parameters are not defined. Additionally, your firm has <u>no quality data records</u> to show that suppliers are being monitored."*

Now as many of the readers already know, Dr. D loves to pontificate about regulatory compliance and the need to have documented evidence to support claims of compliance. In fact, Dr. D's rants on compliance have often been equated to an *"irascible"* (look-it-up) old guy. But hey, the doctor is just attempting to keep the readers out of FDA Purgatory. Enjoy.

Failure to Define

If you decide to pick-up a copy of the QSR or access a copy through www.fda.gov you just might stumble across the frequent use of the phrase *"shall establish."* Shall establish means you had better start pecking away on your computer key board as written procedures are required. If the requirement is not defined in a written procedure, then the device manufacturer can expect to receive a Form 483 observation that commences with the phrase "failure to define." Now if you want to complicate the issue of compliance, do not bother to collect records (a.k.a. documented evidence) to support claims of compliance. One of Dr. D's favorite quotes is; "If an event or activity is not documented in writing, in the eyes of FDA, it never happened." As you can quickly ascertain from the warning letter excerpt in the previous section, this device manufacture not only failed to define but failed to have quality data records. The real travesty is that supplier quality should be one of the easier QSR requirements to achieve compliance. The doctor has taken the liberty to cut and paste the requirement. So why does Dr. D think this requirement is a proverbial cakewalk? Simply stated, create a reasonably coherent procedure, execute to the procedure's content, and keep records to support claims of compliance. Remember, nowhere in §820.50 does it state device manufacturers must spend mega bucks performing on-site audits of suppliers. Establish a system and procedure that is effective for your organization and collect records that reflect compliance. You never want to be the firm that "fails to define or fails to have quality data records."

§820.50 Purchasing Controls

Each manufacturer shall establish and maintain procedures to ensure that all purchased or otherwise received product and services conform to specified requirements.

(a) Evaluation of suppliers, contractors, and consultants. Each manufacturer shall establish and maintain the requirements, including quality requirements that must be met by suppliers, contractors, and consultants. Each manufacturer shall:

(1) Evaluate and select potential suppliers, contractors, and consultants on the basis of their ability to meet specified requirements, including quality requirements. The evaluation shall be documented.

(2) Define the type and extent of control to be exercised over the product, services, suppliers, contractors, and consultants, based on the evaluation results.

(3) Establish and maintain records of acceptable suppliers, contractors, and consultants.

Takeaways

For this chapter, the doctor will leave the readers with two takeaways. One – if the QSR states *"Shall Establish"* that means the FDA is expecting a written procedure. Two – without quality records, there is no chance in Hades of convincing an FDA inspector of compliance during a friendly FDA inspection.

"Shall establish means you had better start pecking away on your computer key board as written procedures are required!"

The Device History Record

The Device History Record

Folks, if an event or activity is not documented in writing, it never happened in the eyes of our friends at FDA. When it comes to retaining accurate records reflecting manufacturing in accordance with the Device Master Record (DMR), having an accurate Device History Record (DHR) to reflect compliance is a salient requirement. In fact, similar to the DMR, the FDA feels so strongly about the DHR the Quality System Regulation (QSR) has a stand-alone requirement for DHR content. Simply stated, the DHR reflects compliance to the DMR, which is a requirement of the QSR, required by FDA. DMR, DHR, QSR, and FDA, enough acronyms for you? Remember, failure to comply with any part of the QSR and the Chief Jailable Officer (CJO) will be wishing for that magic elixir to achieve a "*lenitive*" (look-it-up) effect, as the FDA's response to compliance issues will be harsh. Just to show the readers how serious FDA is about the DHR, Dr. D has taken the liberty of extracting one of the observations from a recently issued warning letter that reflects a violation of 820.184. In fact, it was the very first warning letter the doctor reviewed in support of this chapter's guidance. Note: Dr. D purposely redacted the name of the violating manufacturer to protect the guilty.

FDA Warning Letter Issued on June 12, 2013

Failure to maintain device history records (DHRs). Each manufacturer shall establish and maintain procedures to ensure that DHRs for each batch, lot, or unit are maintained to demonstrate that the device is manufactured in accordance with the device master record and the requirements of this part, as required by 21 CFR 820.184.

For example: Your firm does not have written procedures that govern which documents and information should be present in each DHR. Also, DHRs do not contain a final release signature of the person authorized to release each lot for distribution.

820.184 – Device History Record

Each manufacturer shall maintain device history records (DHR's). Each manufacturer shall establish and maintain procedures to ensure that DHR's for each batch, lot, or unit are maintained to demonstrate that the device is manufactured in accordance with the DMR and the requirements of this part. The DHR shall include, or refer to the location of, the following information:

(a) The dates of manufacture;

(b) The quantity manufactured;

(c) The quantity released for distribution;

(d) The acceptance records which demonstrate the device is manufactured in accordance with the DMR;

(e) The primary identification label and labeling used for each production unit; and

(f) Any device identification(s) and control number(s) used.

Device History Record (DHR)

Let the doctor begin by stating device manufacturers cannot offload their quality and regulatory responsibilities to their suppliers. If a device manufacturer is employing a contract manufacturer in Katmandu, they better be receiving, reviewing, and approving the DHR compiled by the contract manufacturer, including authorizing the release of finished medical devices. On another note, you just might want to visit your contract manufacturer from time-to-time.

Additionally, compiling a DHR is not rocket science. However, some intelligence is required when creating a manufacturing traveler that will become the bulk of the DHR content. Over the previous few chapters, the doctor has climbed to the top of his quality pulpit and pontificated on the importance of Identification, Traceability, and the DMR. For this chapter, it is time for Dr. D to pontificate over the DHR. One thing to keep in mind is that your friends from the agency will eventually stop by for that friendly cup of coffee and an inspection. During that inspection, they will ask to see DMRs and eventually review DHRs to verify finished medical devices are being properly manufactured, in accordance with the DMR.

Dr. D has seen all kinds of DHRs; and there is no secret sauce or magic recipe for creating a great DHR. In fact, the DHR can easily be tailored to a device manufacturer's specific needs, providing all of the information required by §820.184 is included in the DHR. So what needs to be captured in the DHR? The DHR will contain:

- The lot/batch number (or serial number if applicable);

- A reference to each of the procedures used;

- A reference to each of the inspection and test procedures used;

- The names of individuals performing each of the process steps and the dates the process steps were performed;

- The quantity manufactured (pass/fail);

- The quantity released to distribution;

- The name of the individual (could be the CJO) responsible for releasing the lot/batch for distribution; and

- A label retain from the product/package labeling used.

Another important fact to keep in mind and a practice to instill in all employees is another favorite Dr. D acronym, GDP! No one, including the FDA investigators, wants to spend hours stumbling through a DHR review because the GDP is horrendous. Dr. D recognizes that his penmanship is horrible so it was never a good idea for the doctor to make entries into the DHR. Thank God for whiteout correction fluid, just kidding. Make sure, everyone in the organization tasked with making entries in shop floor paperwork, a.k.a., production travelers, exhibits reasonable GDP.

Takeaways

For this chapter's guidance, the doctor will leave the readers with three takeaways. One – make sure your organization scripts a stand-alone procedure for a DHR. Make sure the procedure includes all of the requirements delineated within §820.184. Two – during a friendly visit from the agency, the investigator will get around to reviewing your organization's DHRs. Make sure the DHR reflects that devices were manufactured in accordance with the DMR. Three – neatness and accuracy count so make sure your organization loses the whiteout and trains all employees to GDP.

"If an event or activity is not documented in writing, it never happened in the eyes of our friends at FDA!"

Accurate DHRs are Never Optional

Accurate DHRs are Never Optional

For this Chapter's Devine Guidance, Dr. D is going to briefly expand on the last chapter's topic and the need for device manufacturers to collect, assemble, and retain a Device History Record (DHR) that accurately reflects the complete lot history for finished medical devices. Remember, the DHR is not a nice-to-have or a record to be taken lightly. In fact, the FDA feels so strongly about the importance and composition of the DHR, the Quality System Regulation (21 CFR, Part 820) contains a section dedicated to the almighty DHR (§820.184). If a device manufacturer fails to recognize the importance of the DHR, try managing your organization's complaint management system, performing a complaint investigation, filing an MDR, or even attempting to manage a RECALL (Dr. D's favorite 6-letter word), if accurate lot/batch information is not collected and maintained. In an effort to reduce the doctor's *"sesquipedalian"* (look-it-up) prose, Dr. D will simply state; "Not having a DHR is a bad thing." Enjoy!

Device History Record

So what is the real value of the DHR? For starters, the DHR is the receptacle of documented evidence that each manufactured device, batch, or lot of devices has been manufactured in accordance with the Device Master Record (DMR). Without documented evidence, it will be an impossible task, for the Chief Jailable Officer (CJO) to sit across from an investigator from the agency, and defend the practice of not having adequate DHRs. So the doctor is perfectly clear on his position pertaining the importance of the DHR; **"No DHR will equate to a Form 483 observation, no questions asked."** As a minimum, the DHR shall include:

1. The actual date(s) a device, batch, or lot was manufactured;

2. The actual quantity of devices manufactured;

3. The actual quantity of devices accepted and entered into distribution;

4. All of the records, inspection results, test results, evidence of sterilization, and other quality and manufacturing records that support devices being manufactured in accordance with the DMR;

5. A copy of the actual product label (pouch and carton) and the Directions for Use (DFU); and

6. Any additional identification, serial, or control numbers employed.

Takeaways

Remember, a good rule of thumb is to ensure all documentation relating to the actual manufacturing of a finished medical device be retained in the DHR. Why? Time for a Dr. D broken-record moment; "The DHR is the documented evidence needed, by device manufacturers, to support compliance to the QSR." Why? Because documented evidence is always a device manufacturer's best defense during an FDA inspection. Why? Device manufacturers do not like responding to Form 483 observations. Why? Dr. D says so.

"The DHR is not a nice-to-have or a record to be taken lightly!"

The Device Master Record

The Device Master Record

Ladies and gentlemen, in this chapter's guidance, Dr. D is going to discuss a terrible trend he is starting to see among device manufacturers, the failure to maintain the Device Master Record (DMR) or in some cases the complete failure to create one. Let the doctor begin by stating the FDA believes that the DMR is such an important record, it has its own section under 21 CFR, Part 820 – Subpart M (Records). In fact, Dr. D struggles to understand how a device manufacturer can actually manufacture a device without an accurate DMR. Yes, Dr. D clearly understands that with technology and creativity anything is possible. However, the agency is unwilling to ponder the possibilities so investigators are issuing Form 483 Observations for failing to comply with §820.181 (Device Master Record). In some cases, the failure to comply with §820.181 is finding its way into warning letters, a nice attention grabbing tool employed by FDA. It's the agency's equivalent of: "CAN YOU HEAR ME NOW?" Folks, you have to remember, compliance to the FDA's Quality System Regulation (QSR) is not rocket science. In fact, compliance is rather *"prosaic"* (look-it-up) but a necessary evil if you want to enter medical devices into commerce in the United States. Enjoy!

§820.181 – Device Master Record

Each manufacturer shall maintain device master records (DMR's). Each manufacturer shall ensure that each DMR is prepared and approved in accordance with 820.40. The DMR for each type of device shall include, or refer to the location of, the following information:

(a) Device specifications including appropriate drawings, composition, formulation, component specifications, and software specifications;

(b) Production process specifications including the appropriate equipment specifications, production methods, production procedures, and production environment specifications;

(c) Quality assurance procedures and specifications including acceptance criteria and the quality assurance equipment to be used;

(d) Packaging and labeling specifications, including methods and processes used; and

(e) Installation, maintenance, and servicing procedures and methods.

Excerpt from May 27, 2013 FDA Warning Letter

Failure to maintain adequate device master records, as required by 21 CFR 820.181. For example, the device master records for your manual, half-powered, and full-powered wheelchairs are incomplete because they do not include or refer to the location of production procedures. Your firm has not established procedures for the assembly of manual wheelchair (Model #SS-1) with folding frame; assembly of half-powered wheelchair (Model #HPS-2); assembly of full-powered wheelchair (Model #PS-2); and welding of the frame, and armrest assembly.

Device Master Record

There are two ways of skinning the proverbial cat when it comes to DMR creation. One – you can actual assemble all of the appropriate documentation and place it into a DMR (electronically or paper copy). Two – a simple pointer document can be created that identifies all of the DMR documents and their locations (once again, electronically or paper). See, this really isn't rocket science, so how come device manufacturers are struggling with this requirement?

The next step toward complying with §820.181 is correctly identifying all documents needing to be captured in the DMR. Now if you can read, and the doctor is going to climb out on the limb and assume that if you made it this far into this chapter's guidance you probably can, the documents are actually listed in §820.181. How dare the agency trick everyone and actually provide the information they want device manufacturer's to document and employ. For those of you that are too lazy to read through boring stuff, like regulations, Dr. D will list out the documents that are typically placed into the DMR.

- Device Specifications (including all applicable drawings, composition and formulation)

- Component Specifications

- Software Specifications

- Production Process Specifications (including equipment specifications, production methods, production procedures, and production environment specifications, e.g. ISO 14644-1, Class 7)

- Quality Assurance Procedures (including acceptance criteria and measuring and monitoring equipment to be used)

- Packaging and Labeling Specifications (including all methods and processes employed)

- Installation Procedures and Methods

- Maintenance Procedures and Methods

- Servicing Procedures and Methods

Finally, do not forget to maintain the DMR. For example, if the packaging modality changes from a Poly-Tyvek pouch to a breather bag, you need to ensure this information actually makes it into the DMR. The same holds true for component changes, process changes, and anything else that is used to manufacture the finished medical device, minus the operators of course.

Takeaways

For this chapter's guidance, Dr. D will leave the readers with two takeaways. One – you must have a DMR so just go ahead and create one. Two – once the DMR has been assembled, do not forget to update it. For those of you blessed with electronic document control and data management systems, the task of keeping a DMR current should be a

relatively benign task.

"The FDA believes that the DMR is such an important record, it has its own section under 21 CFR, Part 820 – Subpart M (Records)!"

The Design History File

The Design History File

Dr. D has noticed a disturbing trend, device manufacturers failing to establish a Design History File (DHF). Seriously folks, the doctor is having great difficulty in fathoming how the manufacturer of medical devices does not understand the concept of establishing a DHF. Considering the amount of work required in support of compiling a 510(k) or a PMA submission, the doctor's assumption is that some of the supporting documentation would be extracted from the DHF. In fact, the entire design and development process should be using a DHF as the primary receptacle for the collection of all design and development activities. Can you say documented evidence? You see, the FDA considers the DHF documented evidence that a medical device was designed and developed in accordance with §820.30. If documented evidence does not exist, the FDA will issue a Form 483 observation or in the case of Meridian Medical Systems, a warning letter.

Subpart C - - Design Controls

Sec. 820.30

*(j) **Design history file**. Each manufacturer shall establish and maintain a DHF for each type of device. The DHF shall contain or reference the records necessary to demonstrate that the design was developed in accordance with the approved design plan and the requirements of this part.*

FDA Warning Letter – Meridian Medical Systems (03 July 2013)

In the case of Meridian Medical Systems, the FDA decided that a famous Monopoly move was in order; *"Do not pass go and do not collect your $200!"* In an effort to further *"**ingratiate**"* (look-it-up) their organization with the agency, Meridian provided a vague response to the Form 483 observation. That being said, the FDA's warning letter stated:

> *These violations include, but are not limited to, the following:*
>
> 1. *Failure to establish a design history file, as required by 21 CFR 820.30(j). Specifically,*
>
>   *Your firm does not have a design history file (DHF) for the Meridian DR 200 single panel X-ray system. The system is comprised of a workstation, flat panel detectors, acquisition software and X-ray hardware. Missing elements of the DHF include:*
>
>   - *A design plan for the project*
>   - *Established or approved design inputs/outputs for the system*
>   - *Verification or Validation testing for the system*
>   - *Design Transfer*
>   - *Risk Management for the system*
>   - *Design Reviews.*

If you haven't figured out by now, it is Dr. D's humble opinion the DHF is an immensely important collection of records. As previously stated, the DHF is the receptacle for all documentation associated with the entire design and development process, including design changes made after design transfer. Besides, the FDA will ask to see the DHFs during one of their friendly visits. A well-constructed DHF is always the best friend, although an *"inanimate"* (look-it-up) one, of the quality and regulatory professionals sitting across from the FDA during establishment inspections.

Documentation placed into the DHF should include (not an all-inclusive list):

1. Design & Development Plan;

2. Market Specification;

3. Product Specification;

4. Verification Protocols;

5. Validation Protocols;

6. All Procedures Defining the Design & Development Process;

7. Design Reviews;

8. Test Reports;

9. Drawings;

10. Specifications;

11. Bill of Materials;

12. Routers;

13. Subsequent Design and Process Changes; and

14. All remaining Documentation related Device Design and Development.

Organizations that fail to create and/or maintain a DHF risk suffering through the same fate of Meridian Medical Systems, a Form 483 observation and a subsequent warning letter.

Takeaways

For this chapter's guidance, the doctor will leave the readers with two takeaways. One – the DHF is a salient requirement of the design control so best industry practice is to create one at the start of the design and development process. Two – make sure you treat the DHF as the ultimate receptacle for the collection of *"documented evidence"* for all design and development activities. Remember, the FDA will ask to see and perform a review of the DHF during one of their friendly establishment inspections.

"The FDA considers the DHF documented evidence that a medical device was designed and developed in accordance with §820.30!"

Good Documentation Practices

Good Documentation Practices

Folks - for this chapter Dr. D is going to dive into a topic that can quickly result in a Form 483 observation from my dear friends from FDA or a nonconformance from your well-paid notified bodies. Good Document Practices (GDP) continues to be problematic for device manufacturers and their suppliers. For example, if a device manufacturer starts with a batch size of 100 catheters and during the manufacturing process three (3) catheters fail testing, while an additional two (2) fail mechanical inspection; the remaining quantity to be shipped to sterilization will not be 98. That number folks should be 95. Yes, the doctor knows that some of the readers are laughing; however, these types of errors occur more frequently than many of you may think. Another area where Dr. D frequently sees issues is neatness. People, just like grade school and the fear of Sister "Mad Dog" Mary's ruler smashing down across your knuckles, neatness counts. Please have your manufacturing and quality folks slow down when making entries into production travelers, test reports, and inspection reports. GDP, in Dr. D's humble opinion, is so important it could seriously "*encumber*" (look-it-up) a device manufacturer's success during FDA inspections and notified body audits. That being said, the doctor hopes you enjoy this chapter's guidance.

GDP – Neatness and Accuracy Count

For starters, Dr. D strongly recommends that all device manufacturers have a basic training program for GDP. GDP training should be part of the initial employee orientation, with a refresher course given annually. Why? Because GDP continues to be one of the most frequently cited issues noted during one of the doctor's internal or supplier audits. If Dr. D is seeing GDP as a problem you can bet your organization's last dollar on the fact that FDA and the notified bodies are seeing similar issues. Heck you will actually be doubling that dollar and become a profit center for your organization.

Here are a few additional steps that device manufacturers can take to preclude any chance of receiving a nonconformance from your notified body or a Form 483 observation from the FDA, for bad GDP.

1. As previously stated, training is imperative. Please ensure the results of all training are documented. Why? Because if the training is not documented, then in the eyes of FDA, it never occurred. Can you say documented evidence?

2. Create a written procedure that defines your organization's GDP practices. For example; (a) use of white-out correction fluid is prohibited; (b) define how changes are made, e.g., a single-line drawn through the change/correction; (c) initialing of all changes/corrections; and (d) dating all changes/corrections.

3. Best practice is to annotate all changes/corrections with an actual reason for the change (Reference Figure 1.0).

Figure 1.0 – Using an Annotation to Correct Error

Example: Access Time: *~~2.34~~   3.24 seconds
* Error in recording results CJD 06/03/13

4. All entries made in a report, when recording test data, when recording inspection data, when recording results in the production lot traveler, etc. must always be legible. Remember, neatness counts; otherwise, the Doctor will turn Sister "Mad Dog" Mary loose on your organization (note: she is still alive).

5. Never leave blank spaces in a report, when recording test data, when recording

inspection data, when recording results in the production lot traveler, etc. When using an N/A always remember to date and initial each N/A (Reference Figure 2.0).

Figure 2.0 – Using N/A

Example: Access Time: N/A   CJD 06/03/13

6. If red-line changes are made in support of a pending change to a document or form, always make the change employing red-ink. Make sure that the pending document change order (DCO) number is referenced (Reference Figure 3.0)

Figure 3.0 – Red-Line Changes

Example: Cut catheter to ~~105~~ cm total length change to: 95 cm CJD 06/03/13 – DCO 13-03

Now Dr. D knows that the practical application of GDP sounds pretty easy; however, you would be surprised by the number of organizations that fail to master the art of GDP. Just like anything else, reinforcement of GDP and constant practice makes GDP a non-issue.

Takeaways

For this chapter's guidance, the doctor will leave the readers with just two fundamental takeaways. One – ensure that employees actually receive GDP training. Make sure the training is documented. Why? Because documented evidence is a quality professional's best friend during an FDA inspection or a notified body audit. Two – take the time and actually script a written procedure for GDP. It does not have to be more than two or three pages. In fact, employ the KISS factor (Keep It Simple Stupid).

"GDP continues to be problematic for device manufacturers and their suppliers!"

Identification & Traceability

Identification & Traceability

In this chapter, Dr. D is going to tackle an often overlooked topic by device manufactures, Identification and Traceability. In fact, many device manufacturers completely ignore establishing high-level procedures for Identification and Traceability and attempt to nestle the requirements into a variety of material handling, production control procedures, and work instructions. Guess what, this approach is absolutely driving FDA investigators and notified body auditors completely bonkers. Now please hear the old doctor out, I am not saying it is not ok to place granularity specific to identification and traceability into procedures and work instructions, Dr. D is saying to take the time and create a high-level SOP to address the requirement from a regulatory vantage point. At the end of the day, you will be thanking Dr. D as this approach facilitates smooth inspections and audits. Remember the doctor has never been accused of being quiet or "*demure*" (look-it-up) so when Dr. D strongly recommends that a procedure should be scripted specifically for Identification and Traceability, just do it! The doctor hopes you enjoy this chapter's guidance.

Subpart F – Identification & Traceability

§820.60 Identification

Each manufacturer shall establish and maintain procedures for identifying product during all stages of receipt, production, distribution, and installation to prevent mix-ups.

§820.65 Traceability

Each manufacturer of a device that is intended for surgical implant into the body or to support or sustain life and whose failure to perform when properly used in accordance with instructions for use provided in the labeling can be reasonably expected to result in a significant injury to the user shall establish and maintain procedures for identifying with a control number each unit, lot, or batch of finished devices and where appropriate components. The procedures shall facilitate corrective action. Such identification shall be documented in the DHR.

ID & Traceability

So what in the heck does an Identification and Traceability procedure need to contain? Let's start with the identification of a process for assigning lot/batch (note: lot and batch are typically considered to have the same meaning) numbers upon material receipt. The good news is that most MRP systems have the capability of doing this upon receipt. Make sure that the Bill of Materials (BOMs) employed for assembling kits needed for production are accurate and contain actual material lot numbers. When shop floor paper work is created for finished medical devices (i.e., production travelers or routers) ensure that this documentation also has a unique lot number. Remember the expectation is that traceability for finished medical devices be maintained from the finished device back to raw materials employed in the manufacture of the device. This is specifically true for implantable devices. For manufacturers of capital equipment, e.g., radiotherapy systems, a serial number is usual employed as the system identifier. However, traceability for critical components is required back to the lot number.

Another important aspect of a functioning identification and traceability system is the identification of conforming/acceptable materials, lots, and systems versus nonconforming materials, lots, and systems. It is never a good idea to have accepted and rejected materials in the same general location. Dr. D recommends have a quarantine location (preferably locked) for all nonconforming location. Another valuable tool is line clearance. It is imperative that effective line clearance practices be employed through all aspects of production. Remember, mixing parts and lots is always a bad thing. Guess what? Without effective line clearance, it is just a matter of time when the wrong components, adhesives, or even expired adhesives will be used. It happens and without effective line clearance practices it will continue to happen.

So why is Identification and Traceability so darned important? Well if one has to ask the question, one has not been in industry for too terribly long. Can you say Recall (Dr. D's favorite 6-letter word)? You see, Dr. D's old Irish pal Mr. Murphy is alive and well, living in the medical device industry. Mr. Murphy's ongoing presence ensures that there will be occasional issues with medical device that make them less safe and effective. If a medical device starts hurting patients and/or users, the manufacturers must quickly act to remove suspect product from the market place. If the problem can be traced to a specific device lot or a specific component lot, the recall activities and subsequent recovery of product can be very specific, which results in reduced exposure for the device manufacturer. However, if product identification and traceability has been poor, then it's game over. The device manufacturer will need to recall all products. The fiscal impact and pending loss of market share can be devastating to an organizations bottom line, while resulting in a windfall for their competitors.

Takeaways

For this chapter's guidance, Dr. D will leave the readers with one takeaway. Instead of attempting to rationalize why your current approach to identification and traceability is acceptable, just bite the bullet and script a high-level SOP. For those of you that have invested the time and generated such a procedure, you can pass go and collect your $200.00. For those of you that are still discussing the finer points of identification and traceability, what are you waiting for? It is time to stop talking and start typing.

"Many device manufacturers completely ignore establishing high-level procedures for Identification and Traceability and attempt to nestle the requirements into a variety of material handling, production control procedures, and work instructions!"

Receiving Inspection

Receiving Inspection

Folks, this chapter, the doctor is going to dive into an area that I always struggle with as I see limited value and significant expense; however, it is often a necessary evil, Receiving Inspection (RI). Now don't laugh, but seriously, as an old quality guy Dr. D really does not see much upside in the value of RI. In fact, considering device manufacturers are spending good money for their raw materials, the expectation should be that suppliers produce good products all of the time. Unfortunately, that type of quality utopia still does not exist, as Mr. Murphy is alive and well and living at a supplier near you. Before the doctor jumps into this chapter's guidance, the Dr. D recalls fondly a comment made by Kim Trautman, the FDA's foremost Quality System Regulation expert. According to Trautman; "***Suppliers providing defective products are directly related to an increase in medical device recalls*** (The Sheet – Medical Device Quality Control - May 2007). The "***burgeoning***" (look-it-up) costs associated with playing in the medical device sandbox, continues to escalate. As a result, RI is becoming a less and less attractive alternative; however, if the quality of a supplier is less than stellar, RI becomes a necessary evil. Enjoy this chapter's guidance.

Now for you naysayers out there that do not believe that regulatory bodies never spend much time assessing RI, Dr. D has bridge to sell, the Tobin Bridge. But first, the doctor is going to share a tiny little piece of FDA information known as a warning letter.

Excerpt from May 23, 2013 FDA Warning Letter

*Failure to inspect, test, or otherwise verify that incoming product conforms to specified requirements, as required by 21 CFR 820.80(b). Specifically, **incoming lots** of latex* *tips were not properly inspected, tested, or verified to ensure that they* **conformed** *to specified* **requirements**. *For example;*

a. Latex tip lot 25071 was accepted for use in production on August 22, 2011 despite having more defects than the documented reject level size. The "Latex Tips: Acceptance Testing Worksheet" for lot 25071 documents a total of nine defects and your reject level size was identified as **(b)(4)**.

b. Test results for incoming acceptance of latex tips are not routinely documented. Test results for **(b)(4)** *observed to be missing for lots PJL12/25343 and 25377/POC12.*

We **reviewed** *your firm's* **response** *and conclude that it is* **not adequate**. *Specific test results need to be recorded. Placing an "x" mark only if the test is not within limits is not acceptable. Proper disposition of material not meeting pre-determined specifications cannot be determined at this time and will need to be verified during a subsequent inspection.*

As you can ascertain for yourself, the agency is looking at RI, they are writing Form 483 observations, and if they do not like the response, a Warning Letter is being issued. That being said, the doctor will dive into some of the dynamics of an effective RI program.

Receiving Inspection

If you are still reading this chapter's guidance, the doctor is going to climb out on that limb and assume you either are performing RI or contemplating performing RI. Never fear, the doctor is here. Dr. D will provide some insight into a few salient elements associated with a viable approach to RI.

Sampling and Reduced Inspection

First off, if you must inspect your organization's purchased product, the doctor suggests at least employing a sampling plan (recommend C=0) to reduce the inspection burden. Additionally, Dr. D recommends identifying all of the dimensions/features on the specification as:

- \<C\> - Critical, e.g., AQL 0.40;

- \<M\> Major, e.g., AQL 1.0;

- \<m\> Minor, e.g., AQL 4.0; and

- \<A\> Audit, e.g., one piece.

If the quality being received from your supplier is good, the sampling plan can be loosened. If the quality from you supplier is not so good, you can tighten the sampling, while you begin the search for a new supplier. If the quality is excellent, you may want to consider skip-lot-inspection.

Supplied Data Program

An even better approach to RI is to have your suppliers perform the inspection and provide the statistical data for your review. A program that many organizations call supplied data is premised on a signed agreement between the procuring organization and their supplier. The agreement identifies the features to be inspected, the sampling plan, and the acceptable CpK. For example, the OD for a hypo-tube may be specified at 0.50" +/- 0.01; with a sample size of n=30; and a minimum CpK of 1.33. Statistical data associated with this dimension would be provided with the shipment. Upon receipt, RI personnel will quickly verify the data and move the parts into stock. However, it is strongly recommended that lots be stopped once or twice a year just to keep the suppliers honest, remember Mr. Murphy is alive and well. Since the suppliers are the product experts, they can help you identify the features that require monitoring to ensure compliance with your specification. Typically, two or three dimensions are all that will be required.

First Article Inspection

One of the values Dr. D does see in RI is First Article Inspection (FAI). Performing FAI provides significant value especially in support of product development. An effective approach to FAI can assist the R & D engineers in developing and qualifying components and materials, that when they are assembled into a finished medical device, will be safe and effective in their intended use. Dr. D strongly recommends that all suppliers of custom components and product be required to pass an FAI before shipping production parts. In fact, FAI should be performed prior to placing a supplier into a supplied data program.

Source Inspection

Finally, if your organization is struggling with the quality of product coming from critical suppliers, source inspection may be an option, although a rather expensive one. If a high-dollar-value product is continuing to be inspected, rejected and returned to the supplier, then source inspection can be used to break the cycle, while sending a strong message to the supplier that they inhale greatly (a.k.a., they suck).

Takeaways

As Dr. D stated in the intro to this chapter's guidance, RI can be an expensive proposition. The doctor would much prefer that the supplier take some ownership in the product, material, or service they are providing. However, the device industry is far from perfect, including the suppliers. That being said, the doctor will leave just one takeaway from this chapter's guidance. If your organization decides to pursue and RI program, jump into the deep end of the pool with both feet and do not be afraid of getting wet. What in the heck does that mean Dr. D? It means make sure the RI personnel are adequately trained, the program (supported by a written procedure) has provisions for: (a) sampling plans, including reduced and tightened inspection; (b) supplied data; (c) FAI; (d) source inspection; and (e) demolition support for making bad suppliers disappear (just kidding about the demolition piece, a simple disqualification will do).

"Remember, Mr. Murphy is alive and well and living at a supplier near you!"

The Importance of Calibration

The Importance of Calibration

While perusing through the FDA's warning letter database, I was astounded to find a manufacturer that was not calibrating their monitoring and measuring devices. People, this is the 21st Century and if a device manufacturer has not figured out that gages need to be calibrated and traceable to a national standard, e.g. NIST, then the device manufacturer is probably in the wrong business. Just maybe the manufacturing of flyswatters might be a viable option. Seriously, Inspection, Measuring, and Test Equipment (§820.72) or its ISO cousin Control of Monitoring and Measuring Devices (ISO 13485:2003, Clause 7.6) have been industry mainstays for years. The Quality System Regulation (QSR) and ISO 13485 are quite similar in that device manufacturers **shall** establish a written procedure or procedures; and equipment is expected to be calibrated and records associated with the calibration **shall be** retained. Sorry folks, a regulation or standard just does not get any easier to understand then the requirements surrounding calibration. That being said, the doctor hopes that use find this chapter's guidance "*utile*" (look-it-up).

FDA Warning Letter Issued on June 20, 2013

Failure to ensure that all inspection, measuring, and test equipment, including mechanical, automated, or electronic inspection and test equipment, is suitable for its intended purposes and is capable of producing valid results, as required by 21 CFR 820.72(a). For example, your firm did not calibrate gauges, thermometers, and other devices used to monitor the (b)(4) manufacturing process for the (b)(4).

The doctor has taken the opportunity to cut-and-paste the requirement from the QSR so the readers can focus on this chapter's guidance. Basically, the FDA, through the

QSR, conveys one very clear message; "Device manufacturers must calibrate equipment (as appropriate) and collect records to support claims of compliance.

21 CFR, Part 820.72 – Inspection, Measuring, and Test Equipment

(a)Control of inspection, measuring, and test equipment. Each manufacturer shall ensure that all inspection, measuring, and test equipment, including mechanical, automated, or electronic inspection and test equipment, is suitable for its intended purposes and is capable of producing valid results. Each manufacturer shall establish and maintain procedures to ensure that equipment is routinely calibrated, inspected, checked, and maintained. The procedures shall include provisions for handling, preservation, and storage of equipment, so that its accuracy and fitness for use are maintained. These activities shall be documented.

(b)Calibration. Calibration procedures shall include specific directions and limits for accuracy and precision. When accuracy and precision limits are not met, there shall be provisions for remedial action to reestablish the limits and to evaluate whether there was any adverse effect on the device's quality. These activities shall be documented.

(1)Calibration standards. Calibration standards used for inspection, measuring, and test equipment shall be traceable to national or international standards. If national or international standards are not practical or available, the manufacturer shall use an independent reproducible standard. If no applicable standard exists, the manufacturer shall establish and maintain an in-house standard.

(2)Calibration records. The equipment identification, calibration dates, the individual performing each calibration, and the next calibration date shall be documented. These records shall be displayed on or near each piece of equipment or shall be readily available to the personnel using such equipment and to the individuals responsible for calibrating the equipment.

Calibration

Let Dr. D begin by saying, the metrology house selected for calibration should be ISO/IEC 17025:2005 accredited. This requirement should not be negotiable. Obviously, device manufacturers can place the calibration requirement squarely on the backs of employees and calibrate equipment in-house. However, Dr. D has a better idea, find a good metrology lab and outsource the fun. Regardless of where the calibration is performed, device manufacturers still need an SOP to document their approach to managing calibration. As a minimum, the scripted procedure should contain:

- Calibration cycles;

- A process for labeling of pieces of equipment with a calibration sticker that contains: (a) date calibrated; (b) date due; and (c) calibrated by;

- Provisions for managing calibration records;

- Provisions for labeling equipment that is not calibrated (i.e., calibration not required or for reference only);

- Provisions for identification and removal from service of measuring and monitoring equipment when calibration has expired or the equipment is damaged;

- Handling, preservation and storage of equipment;

- A provision for reviewing the calibration report if an independent metrology facility is employed for calibration;

- A traceability requirement to a national standard, e.g. NIST; and

- Provisions for pursing corrective action if a piece of equipment is found to be out-of-tolerance during the calibration process, including a notification process.

If a device manufacturer decides to calibrate their equipment, calibration procedures will need to be scripted delineating the calibration process, including accuracy and tolerances for each type of gage or equipment. As the doctor previously stated, it may be more practical to just outsource the calibration. If outsourcing is selected as the preferred process, make sure you review the calibration report for accuracy and trends versus previous calibration cycles.

Takeaways

For this chapter's guidance, Dr. D will leave the readers with two takeaways. One – it is much easier to outsource calibration to a competent and ISO/IEC 17025:2005 accredited lab. However, if your organization decides to tackle calibration (in-house) then equipment and gage-specific calibration procedures will be required. Two – Regardless of the approach pursued for calibration (in-house versus outsourced) device manufacturers are still required to script a procedure defining the approach to calibration.

"This is the 21st Century and if a device manufacturer has not figured out that gages need to be calibrated and traceable to a national standard, e.g. NIST, then the device manufacturer is probably in the wrong business!"

Internal Audits

Internal Audits

Listen up people, the doctor is growing tired of writing non-conformances for organizations failing to establish a program and procedure for internal audits and actually performing audits. Yes, actually performing audits. Audits are good things and when performed properly, and help organizations ensure their QMS remains in compliance with all of those annoying little thing like regulations and standards.

Not too long ago, in the distant past, in a land not so far away, Dr. D was visiting one of my client's suppliers for the purpose of performing a supplier audit against the requirements delineated within ISO 13485:2003. Now keep in mind the doctor is an old guy so it really takes something outrageous to see the doctor's jaw hit the floor and keep from laughing hysterically. This supplier's quality guru, and I use the term guru loosely, shared their internal audit schedule that eloquently planned for audits to be performed over a two-year period. Unfortunately, audits were not being performed. When the doctor inquired as to why no audits were being performed, the response was a resounding, "We don't have to perform audits we just need to plan for them." Wow (Dr. D still smile when he thinks about this audit)! The quality guru was still arguing when asked to sign the non-conformance form. Needless to say, this auditee treated Dr. D as "*algid*" (look-it-up) as ice during the remainder of the audit debrief. Excuse the doctor, my bad for enforcing compliance. That being said, this chapter's guidance is all about the importance of internal quality audits.

The Requirement

Regardless of the regulatory requirement or standard being driven by: 21 CFR,

Part 820.22 (Quality Audit); Ministerial Ordinance 169 – Article56 (Internal Audit); or ISO 13485:2003, Clause 8.2.2 (Internal Audit), device manufacturers must perform internal audits or outsource the internal audit process to a qualified firm or individual, like Dr. D and Devine Guidance International. Failure to perform internal audits or take appropriate action when issues with the QMS are noted; will result in a Form 483 observation from the FDA and a potential major non-conformance from a device manufacturer's notified body. Just an FYI – these are bad things.

On another note, performing audits late will also get device manufacturers in hot water with Agency, their notified bodies, and other regulatory bodies scattered around the globe. You see, since we are not talking about toys here, but medical devices, the expectation is that medical device manufacturers have the appropriate infrastructure in place to successfully manage the QMS. If audits are not being performed on time, then there just might be a resource issue. Can you say another Form 483 observation or audit nonconformance due to lack of resources or effective management oversight?

Program Construction

An effective internal audit program can be eloquent in its simplicity, so start simple with a written procedure. Since §820.22 does not provide a lot of granularity in regards to an internal audit program, the doctor recommends following ISO 13485 for guidance in regards to content. As a minimum, an internal audit program and/or procedure should contain the following tidbits of information (as appropriate).

- The device manufacturer must publish an audit schedule that reflects audits at planned intervals (yes, it is acceptable to perform all of the audits at once; however, the practice is not extremely effective).

- The internal audits should be driven by importance and results of previous audits (if previous audits uncover weaknesses in the QMS, the frequency of audits in the problem area should probably be increased).

- Make sure the auditor requirements are built into the procedure, i.e., certified quality auditor or specific training requirements (recommend reviewing ISO 19011).

- The audit procedure should contain a requirement for an opening meeting (as needed).

- The audit procedure should contain a requirement for a closing meeting (as needed).

- The audit procedure should contain a requirement for documenting the results of internal audits, including record retention.

- As part of the documentation process it is imperative that the area(s) audited, personnel interviewed, processes reviewed, and procedures reviewed be documented.

- The audit procedure should address the process of pursing corrective action to correct audit deficiencies.

- The audit procedure should contain a clause for performing additional audits, when the results of an audit are unsatisfactory.

- Finally, the results of audits need to find their way into management review, including actions taken to address QMS performance issues.

NOTE: Device manufacturers are not required to share the result of internal audits with FDA. They only have to provide evidence that they have been performed.

Takeaways

Folks the doctor understands audits are time consuming, that is why organizations such as Devine Guidance International come into being. If you do not have the trained resources to perform internal audits, then by all means outsource the process. However, buyers please beware; not all auditing firms or auditors are created equal. In fact, there is;

"The Good, The Bad, and The Ugly when it comes to auditors (sounds like a Clint
Eastwood movies). Regardless of the approach to performing internal quality audits, you
have to complete them and complete them on time.

*"Audits are good things and when
performed properly, and help
organizations ensure their QMS
remains in compliance with all of
those annoying little thing like
regulations and standards!"*

Attributes of a Good Auditor

Attributes of a Good Auditor

Dr. D is going to switch gears this chapter and dive into a topic that is not frequently addressed by writers, the selection and training of quality management system (QMS) auditors. Good auditors are always in demand regardless of if the QMS being evaluated is premised on 21 CFR, Part 820 (FDA's QSR); ISO 13485: 2003; EN ISO 13485:2012; ISO 9001:2008; or AS 9100. Auditors are a unique group of individuals capable of blending intellect, integrity, tenaciousness, humility, a sense of humor, and auditing demeanor (in Dr. D's opinion; "Da meaner, Da better - just kidding).

Additionally, the doctor strongly believes that there is some value in having a certified lead auditor to ride herd over an organization's internal audit program; however, having a lead-auditor certification in every conceivable regulation and standard, not so much. Folks - Dr. D is sorry if his tone is borderline quality sacrilegious when talking about paying for external training; however, there is more value in being out there in the field and actually auditing versus spending an eternity in classrooms. If an organization feels that formal auditor training, formal auditor training, and more formal auditor training will have an overwhelming impact and *"redound"* (look-it-up) on the organization's approach to quality, it is the doctor's belief the money can be better spent elsewhere, like buying a bridge. Did Dr. D mention he is selling the Bay Bridge? Auditors should be adequately trained, and possess the appropriate level of experience and education, period! That being said, Dr. D hopes you enjoy this chapter's brief guidance.

Auditor Requirements

For those of you familiar with ISO 19011:2011, the doctor is sure you are aware that there is no formal requirement for auditors to be certified. If a registrar or notified body states that your auditors must be certified, **PUSH BACK!** If they continue to insist their interpretation of ISO 19011 is correct, ask for a new auditor that actually comprehends applicable standards and regulations. The doctor also strongly suggests that you recommend having the auditor that fails to interpret the certification requirement correctly to **read ISO 19011:2011, Clause 7, all of it!** Did the doctor mention your organizations actually pay registrars and notified bodies for their abuse; excuse me – audit support? ISO 19011 contains some excellent points associated with ensuring auditors have the appropriate level of training and experience.

Imperative Skills, Knowledge, and Personal Attributes

The following bulleted list should not be construed as all inclusive. Dr. D recommends reading ISO 19011 for an all-inclusive list of auditor attributes. However, some of the more important skills, knowledge, and personal attributes associated with a good auditor (the doctor's opinion) are:

- Integrity;
- A good sense of humor;
- Open mindedness;
- A good sense of humor;
- Tactfulness when dealing with people;
- A good sense of humor;

- Observant;

- A good sense of humor;

- Perceptive and capable of comprehending complex systems and processes;

- A good sense of humor;

- Tenacious;

- A good sense of humor;

- Ability to make decisions;

- A good sense of humor;

- Ability to be fair and objective;

- A good sense of humor;

- Able to act independently of others;

- A good sense of humor;

- Interact appropriately and constructively with others;

- A good sense of humor;

- Sensitive to cultural differences;

- A good sense of humor;

- In depth knowledge of quality management systems;

- A good sense of humor;

- Understanding potential statutory requirements impacting an audit;

- A good sense of humor;

- Knowledge of special processes (when deem necessary);

- A good sense of humor;

- Ability to collect and organize evidence of compliance and non-compliance;

- A good sense of humor;

- Appropriate level of education;

- A good sense of humor;

- Good written composition skills;

- A good sense of humor;

- Ability to accurately formulate non-conformances when noted;

- A good sense of humor

- Applicable audit training;

- A good sense of humor

- Practical experience (most important in Dr. D's humble opinion); and

- A good sense of humor.

Did Dr. D mention that auditors really do need to possess a good sense of humor? Levity is great way to break the ice and lower the stress and tension typically associated with an audit.

Is Certification Required?

As previously stated, there is no formal requirement to have auditors and lead auditors certified; however, it would be considered prudent to have at least on certified lead auditor to manage an organization's audit program and to assist with auditor selection and training program. If resources are limited, you can always employ a 3rd-party firm such as Devine Guidance International, Inc. Dr. D would love to have the opportunity to help your organization improve their QMS.

Takeaways

For this edition of DG, the doctor will lead the readers with two takeaways. One – there is no better way to gain the appropriate level of audit experience than actually performing audits. Two – although there is no formal requirement for auditors to be certified, it would be considered prudent to have at least one lead auditor with a current RAB certification (regardless of standard).

"Did the doctor mention your organizations actually pay registrars and notified bodies for their abuse; excuse me – audit support?"

FDA versus the Notified Body

FDA versus the Notified Body

Folks – Dr. D wrote this chapter at 35,000 feet. In this chapter, the doctor is going to provide a brief parody on the little differences and nuances between FDA and your friendly notified bodies. Now the doctor will be the first to admit he is an old guy. That being said, I have fond memories of one of my favorite comedians, the late George Carlin. Years ago, for those that can remember that far back, old George did a very creative comparison between football stadiums and baseball parks. It was hilarious. Although medical device regulatory and quality compliance is often a dry topic, I will attempt to make the comparison between FDA and the notified bodies entertaining. For the notified bodies and members of the agency, please do not take offense with this chapter's as it is just the doctor's attempt at humor. In general, Dr. D hopes the readers are "*sentient*" and appreciative of the doctor's humor. Enjoy and let the comparisons begin.

Viva la Difference

The FDA performs inspections for the purpose of determining compliance to federal regulations; and if necessary, collects evidence that could be used in court. Can you say Form 483 observation? Notified bodies perform audits, identify opportunities for improvement, and issue non-conformances to drive corrective action. If a device manufacturer fails to respond to a Form 483 observation, a warning letter is issued. If a device manufacturer fails to respond to a nonconformance, a courtesy telephone call and subsequent email is sent by the notified body. If a device manufacturer fails to address the warning letter concerns, the FDA can use the Department of Justice and the Federal

Courts to drive compliance. Can you say Consent Decree? Can you name your Chief Jailable Officer (CJO)? If a device manufacture fails to respond to their notified body's request for corrective action, their certificates are suspended and/or revoked. However, kissing and making up with the notified body, including a group hug and a verse of Kumbia, is considerably more forgiving then a smooch with FDA. The agency is far-less forgiving. FDA investigators carry a badge and a few are licensed to carry firearms. The notified body auditor carries a business card. FDA inspections are paid courtesy of the American taxpayer and establishment registration fees. Device manufacturers contract with and pay their notified bodies for the performance of their audits and sometimes, the subsequent pain. The FDA charges an arm and a leg for the review of Pre-Market Approval (PMA) submissions (Class III devices) and a relatively tidy sum for 510(k) submission reviews (Class II devices). In comparison, the notified body review fees are reasonable for Design Dossiers (Class III) devices. Once clearance is received for a Class II or Class III device in the US, it is basically on the market for the life of the device, providing the device continues to be safe and effective and is not racking up the MDRs. In Europe, depending on the notified body, Class III devices must be renewed every three to five years. These reviews are not free. If the devices sold in Europe are racking up the vigilance reports, the Competent Authorities, from impacted Member States, will get involved. Note: the Competent Authorities are starting to bare their teeth and show some fangs. So many more comparisons are possible but the doctor has so little time as the intercom of the Boeing 777 blares out; "Ladies and gentlemen it is time to turn-off and stow your electronic devices."

Takeaways

In closing, the doctor hopes you have found this chapter's brief guidance to be entertaining. If device manufacturers are doing the right things in regards to compliance, then a visit from FDA should never be feared but always respected. As for the notified bodies, they should always be respected; however, if you are not pleased with your notified body, you are always free to change to another.

"For the notified bodies and members of the agency, please do not take offense with this chapter's as it is just the doctor's attempt at humor!"

The Notified Body

Notified Body

Yes the doctor realizes that for the most part notified bodies are a European-centric thing; however, most medical device companies will eventually end up serving the EU market place. Considering the notified bodies actually issue QMS certificates versus the agency's inspection approach, the doctor felt that dedicating a chapter to the notified bodies probably has some merit. Since the beginning of 2013, Dr. D has had the opportunity or let's say misfortune in some cases, of sitting through notified body audits for a my clients or receiving disturbing phone calls from clients about audit issues. Let the doctor begin by stating, you pay for this abuse so your organization might as well get their money's worth. For starters, Dr. D is seeing a recurrence of auditors that just do not understand ISO 13485; ISO 14971; ISO 19011; or even worse 93/42/EEC. How can you be an effective notified body auditor if you do not understand the Medical Device Directive? The doctor is truly seeing the good, the bad, and the ugly when it comes to notified body audits. Before I dive into this chapter's guidance, please remember: "You pay the notified bodies and they work for you." If you do not like the relationship with your notified body, by all means file for that divorce and move on. If you are unhappy with BSI then move to SGS. If SGS is giving you fits, then move to DEKRA. If DEKRA isn't working for you then try TUV-R or UL. If TUV-R or UL is giving your organization severe indigestion then move to BSI. People, you have choices, so just like a marriage pick a notified body that you are comfortable working with or continue to suffer in silence. It's your device company, so it's your pain! For you notified bodies reading this chapter's guidance, remember Dr. D loves you man and would never intentionally *"fustigate"* (look-it-up) your efforts to drive the quality and regulatory compliance of your clients. However, for those notified body auditors making stuff up as you pretend to know what you are doing, the gigs up my friends. It is time for all of you wannabes to move on to another industry, such as an official meet-and-greet person at a big-box store. If that doesn't work, how about trying; "Clean-up on aisle nine." Regardless of choice, if you cannot correctly interpret standards and regulations, you are clearly in the wrong industry. That being said, I hope you enjoy this chapter's guidance.

Flawed Comments/Observations

There is no doubt most auditors possess a plethora of knowledge that they rely on during the course of an audit. Frankly, the doctor's expectation is that auditors have a fundamental understanding of the regulations, standards, and even more important, the processes they are assessing. However, some of the comments and observations I see coming from notified body auditors, frightens this old doctor, especially if the auditees do not push back on such nonsensical non-conformances or perceived requirements. That being said, Dr. D is going to share some of the more egregious comments and findings coming from notified body audits in 2013.

- *Failure to comply with harmonized standards.* Folks, there is no requirements to do so. Harmonized standards are strongly recommended but not mandated by 93/42/EEC, the European Medical Device Directive.

- *The MDD requires that the notified bodies audit all of your suppliers*. Beep, beep, beep; wrong again folks. There is no such requirement just another money maker for the notified bodies. If medical device manufacturers accept this type of comment as a mandated requirement, then the cost of playing in this sand box will quickly escalate. However, if you identify a supplier as crucial or critical, you may be opening yourselves up for unannounced supplier audits (performed by your notified body, at your expense). You have been warned by doctor D.

- *ISO 13485:2003 is no longer a valid standard.* Beep, beep, beep; wrong again. Although EN ISO 13485:2012 has been harmonized; outside of the EU in places such as the United States, ISO 13485:2003 remains a valid standard. In fact, Health Canada specifically references 13485:2003 in SOR/98-282 (The Canadian Medical Device Regulation).

- *It is required that your auditors must be certified by a recognized accreditation board.* Once again, this nonconformance would be incorrect. ISO 19011 requires that auditors be competent, period! Formal certification for all auditors is a noble pursuit; however, it is also an expensive one. Dr. D strongly recommends an in-house training of auditors occur or when in doubt, outsource the entire internal audit program.

- *ISO 9001 requires written procedures in support of all clauses.* Sorry, wrong again. ISO 9001 requires a quality manual and high-level procedures for the following clauses:
    - 4.2.3 Control of Documents
    - 4.2.4 Control of Records;
    - 8.2.2 Internal Audits;
    - 8.3 Control of Nonconforming Product;
    - 8.5.2 Corrective Action; and
    - 8.5.3 Preventive Action.

What can you do?

Folks, the best advice Dr. D can give during an audit is to push back if the nonconformance is not clear or the nonconformance is not valid. Demand that the auditor give you the specific regulation or standards title, clause, section, paragraph, or sentence for which your organization is failing to comply. If the auditor cannot give you the specific requirement, repeat after the doctor: "Your observation is not valid, please move on." If the auditor is persistent in his or her ignorance of a standard or regulation, elevate your concern to the notified body's home office. Remember, you pay for this abuse and deserve to receive a fair assessment based on actual regulations and standards.

Takeaways

The doctor will leave two takeaways from this chapter's guidance. (1) Notified bodies are not created equal nor are their auditors. If you are having issues with a notified body, it is acceptable to change notified bodies. However, depending on the number of products entered into the European device market, changing notified bodies could be an expensive endeavor. (2) Do not be afraid to push back. If you feel the nonconformance is not premised on a regulation or standard or the auditor's interpretation of a regulation or standard is incorrect, call them out and clearly state your concern. If your concern falls on deaf ears, elevate your concern to the notified body's home office.

"Dr. D is seeing a recurrence of auditors that just do not understand ISO 13485; ISO 14971; ISO 19011; or even worse 93/42/EEC!"

Whitepaper on Effective

Supplier Management

Whitepaper on Effective Supplier Management

The medical device industry is in a perpetual state of change as technology continues to evolve, while standards and regulations are in a constant state of rescript to ensure the ongoing safety and efficacy of medical devices. This dynamic industry demands an equally dynamic approach to quality. *"Antediluvian"* (look-it-up) approaches to quality that were premised on inspection, inspection, and more inspection, are no longer viable options. An area of opportunity, that demands serious attention, is the renewed focus on the importance of supplier management in the medical device industry. In recent years, the FDA has increased vigilance in regards to the prevention of medical device manufacturers from inadvertently procuring defective products and the subsequent employment of defective products into finished medical devices. According to Kimberly Trautman, the FDA's current Good Manufacturing Practices (cGMP) and Quality System Regulations (QSR) expert, suppliers providing defective products are directly related to an increase medical device recalls. Because of increased recall activity, effective supplier management tools are needed to mitigate supplier risk.

Devine Guidance for Managing Key Attributes of a FDA-Compliant Quality Management System

Index of Key Terms

Defensive-Receiving Inspection. Defensive-receiving inspection is the inspection performed on materials, after receipt from the supplier, but prior to releasing procured materials into inventory.

First Article Inspection (FAI). An inspection process employed to determine if the initial batches of manufactured devices (internal or external suppliers) meet their specification.

Ppk. Ppk is the statistical term for Process Capability Index. It reflects the *long-term* capability of a process. Additionally, (a) statistical means, (b) upper specification limits, and (c) lower specification limits, are all factors that influencing the calculation for Ppk.

Quality System Regulation (QSR). The Quality System Regulation (QSR) is the widely accepted acronym for 21CFR Part 820, the quality system regulation that all medical device manufacturers must comply with to sell and distribute products in the United States.

Supplier Corrective Action Request (SCAR). A form employed as part of a supplier corrective action to; (a) document a supplier nonconformance, (b) document action pursued to prevent nonconformance recurrence, (c) verify effectiveness of corrective action pursued, and (d) verification of completion of all activities by the issuing organization.

Supplier Statistical Data (SSD). Supplier Statistical data is an inspection program in which a supplier's measurement data is included with each shipment. The supplier performs the out-going inspection, collects the measurement data in a statistical format, and reviews the data for compliance prior to shipment. Upon material receipt, the customer performs a review of the SSD received with the product shipment.

Background

Since early 2010, the doctor has enlisted his colleagues and asked that they read

Dr. D's rants, posted in the weekly blog "Devine Guidance" (The Medical Device

Summit); even if Dr. D's views and opinions appear to be obverse to their own. That

being said, the intent of this chapter is to share with the readers a whitepaper containing

relevant and practical information, extracted from the doctor's weekly column, doctoral

dissertation, previously authored Dr. D books, and research, influencing the medical device industry today; while sharing proven approaches and processes needed for developing an effective approach to supplier-management. Dr. D's intention, as the crazed author, is to highlight key areas where regulatory bodies are beginning to exhibit a keen interest, while providing effective tools needed for effective supplier management in support of the medical device industry.

The first area of opportunity that demands some serious attention is the renewed focus on the importance of supplier management, in the medical device industry, by the FDA. As stated in this chapter's opening paragraph, the agency has increased its vigilance in regards to the prevention of medical device manufacturers from inadvertently procuring non-conforming materials from their suppliers and the subsequent employment of these materials into finished medical devices. The Code of Federal Regulations, Title 21 Part 820, a.k.a., the QSR, requires all medical device manufacturers and medical device distributors to establish a certain level of control over their supplier base, in accordance with Subpart E – Purchasing Controls. The Code of Federal Regulations, under Title 21, Part 820 – Section 820.50, regulates purchased-material controls to ensure the evaluation of suppliers, components, and raw materials occurs prior to the incorporation of procured materials into the manufacturing of medical devices.

There are several key attributes associated with an effective supplier-management system; and because the QSR is not overly prescriptive when it comes to the details of a system, organizations are free to develop systems tailored to their manufacturing and operational environment. Since the vast majority of medical device manufacturers distribute product both inside and outside of the United States, compliance with additional regulations, such as the Medical Device Directive, a.k.a., MDD (93/42/EEC) become additional mandated requirements. Standards such an ISO 13485:2012 must also be considered during the development and implementation of an effective supplier-management system. Additionally, risk is playing an increasingly prevalent role in identifying critical factors associated with supplier selection, defensive-receiving inspection activities pursued, ongoing supplier maintenance, supplier corrective action, etc. Furthermore, business risk, compliance risk, and risk of device failure, premised on supplier performance issues, needs to be adequately identified and woven into the fabric of an effective supplier-management system.

Regulations & Requirements

In this section, you will find the key clauses extracted from the QSR and ISO that define the basic elements needed for a compliant approach to supplier management. A salient concept to remember is supplier management is considered subservient to purchasing and most regulations treat supplier management activities as a subset to procurement.

QSR – Subpart E – Purchasing Controls

Section 820.50

Each manufacturer shall establish and maintain procedures to ensure that all purchased or otherwise received product and services conform to specified requirements.

(a)Evaluation of suppliers, contractors, and consultants. Each manufacturer shall establish and maintain the requirements, including quality requirements, that must be met by suppliers, contractors, and consultants. Each manufacturer shall:

(1) Evaluate and select potential suppliers, contractors, and consultants on the basis of their ability to meet specified requirements, including quality requirements. The evaluation shall be documented.

(2) Define the type and extent of control to be exercised over the product, services, suppliers, contractors, and consultants, based on the evaluation results.

(3) Establish and maintain records of acceptable suppliers, contractors, and consultants.

(c) Purchasing data. Each manufacturer shall establish and maintain data that clearly describe or reference the specified requirements, including quality requirements, for purchased or otherwise received product and services. Purchasing documents shall include, where possible, an agreement that the suppliers, contractors, and consultants agree to notify the manufacturer of changes in the product or service so that manufacturers may determine whether the changes may affect the quality of a finished device. Purchasing data shall be approved in accordance with 820.40.

ISO 13485:2012

7.4 Purchasing

7.4.1 The organization shall establish documented procedures to ensure that purchased product conforms to specified purchase requirements.

- The type and extent of control applied to the supplier and the purchased product shall be dependent upon the effect of the purchased product on subsequent product realization or the final product.

- The organization shall evaluate and select suppliers based on their ability to supply product in accordance with the organization's requirements. Criteria for selection, evaluation, and re-evaluation shall be established. Records of the results of evaluations and any necessary actions arising from the evaluation shall be maintained.

Supplier Selection Process

The first salient concept to remember is an effective selection of a supplier must be requirements driven. Business needs such as; (a) quality, (b) regulatory and compliance, (b) manufacturing capabilities, (c) technology, (d) capabilities (e) customer service, (f) delivery and cycle times, and (g) life-cycle management, are worthy of consideration, as part of the selection process. The second salient concept is risk. The assessment of business risk, regulatory risk, risk of product failure, etc. must be effectively gauged throughout the entire supplier selection process. The third salient concept is the development of an effective supplier survey. Finally, you must remember the importance of documentation, documentation, and more documentation. All of the supplier selection activities must be thoroughly documented, in writing I might add. Why? Because in the eyes of the FDA, notified bodies, and other regulatory bodies, if events are not documented in writing, they just did not happen; and just like grade school accuracy counts.

Requirements Driven Supplier Evaluation Process

You would not buy a house without sharing with your real-estate agent some basic requirements as to what your needs are, i.e., size, rooms, location, etc. Well, guess what? The supplier selection process cannot commence until basic requirements and needs are defined by your organization. For all of you engineers used to working from a napkin drawing, once your ideas are captured and formulated, a formal document really needs to be created, e.g., component specification. Additionally, when defining these requirements the approach pursued must be cross-functional. Yes, engineers are driving the show because they are tasked with owning the design and development. However, quality, regulatory, manufacturing, procurement, materials, supply chain, marketing, etc. are key stakeholders; and should provide input into the selection process. Furthermore, if a candidate supplier possesses a quality system certified by a recognized registrar or notified body, the premise of the initial supplier visit can be focused on process and overall business capabilities. Finally, because developing suppliers and qualifying material is expensive, never let one functional group be the sole stakeholder in the selection process. The final decision to approve and add a supplier to your organization's Approved Supplier's List (ASL) must be a collaborative one.

Risk

For medical device manufacturers, it is incumbent upon the organization to investigate the capabilities of potential suppliers prior to the commencement of an on-site assessment. I strongly recommend starting with the moderately famous and extremely useful D & B, and no, I am not a paid spokesperson for this service. The Dunn & Bradstreet report provides a condensed business synopsis on potential suppliers and can save an organization from much grief and pain if potential suppliers have cash flow issues, pending litigation, or other significant problems that can influence their business both short and long term. Remember; if a potential supplier is experiencing business problems, those problems will quickly become the problem of your organization, if the decision is made to proceed with the relationship. Now I am not implying the D & B should be the all-encompassing selection tool; however, it should carry some weight in regards to the selection process.

The second important factor relating to risk is the potential failure of a procured component and the influence a failed component could have on the finished medical device. I strongly recommend, early in the design and development process, linking the component failure risk back to the design and preferably to the design Failure Mode and Effects Analysis (dFMEA). Additionally, best-in-class industry practices drive the alignment of suppliers into categories premised on risk and organizational need. For example, when selecting a supplier for providing a disposable manufacturing aide such as a finger cot, the selection and evaluation process will differ dramatically from that of a contract manufacturer. The identification of categories and the subsequent placement of suppliers into these categories are dictated by organizational structure and need. An example of a supplier category table is depicted in Table 1. Remember; the table is only an example and not all encompassing model as the final model will be premised on your organizational need.

Table 1 - *Sample Categorization of Suppliers*

Category & Assessment		Applicability
Category 1 • ***Annual On-Site Assessment Mandatory – Due to Risk*** • ***No-Change Agreement*** • ***Quality Agreement***		• OEM's, or Contract Manufacturers
Category 2 • ***On-Site Assessment Mandatory - Premised on Schedule & Risk (3-years)*** • ***No-Change Agreement*** • ***Quality Agreement***		• Components Identified as Critical Premised on the Device FMEA • Sterilization Service Providers • Laboratory Services Providers • Analytical Test Labs • Calibration/Metrology Provider • Notified Bodies
Category 3 • ***On-Site Assessment as Necessary - Premised on Risk*** • ***Mail-In Survey (in lieu of on-site)*** • ***No-Change Agreement*** • ***Quality Agreement***		• Non-Critical Custom Material, Process, and/or Component • Offsite Record Storage • Environmental Services Provider
Category 4 • ***Mail-In Survey Required*** • Current ISO 9001, ISO 13485, or AS 9100 Quality Certificate is acceptable in lieu of survey.		• Standard Catalog Component Manufacturers • Low-Risk Components • Distributors of Catalog Components
Category 5 • *No Requirement for Quality System*		• Transportation Services (UPS, USPS, etc.) • Consultants • Facility Services, i.e., Janitorial Services, Pest Control, etc.

Supplier Assessments Survey

In reviewing multiple types of supplier assessments, as part of Dr. D's doctoral research, one of the shortfalls noted was a strong reliance on a single model by organizations to assess their supplier base. The one-shoe-fits-all approach does not lend itself to being a proactive and efficient approach for effective supplier management. For example, requirements for a contract sterilization supplier will differ from the requirements that are relevant for a machined component supplier. The fundamental quality system requirements may be the same; however, manufacturing processes and inspection methodologies will differ. So how does an organization address the technological differences? Dr. D recommends creating commodity-specific surveys to support the supplier assessment process. Since quality-specific requirements such as corrective and preventive action, non-conforming material, management review, and similar quality processes are standard throughout the medical device industry, a single bank of questions, specific to quality systems, can be created and placed into a dedicated quality section within each survey. These questions would be applicable for all suppliers. Additionally, for a low-risk application, the quality certificate, from a recognized notified body or registrar, should be acceptable in lieu of a supplier survey. Furthermore, not all suppliers will require an on-site assessment, as this approach is expensive. A well-designed supplier quality questionnaire, that captures relevant business and quality information, can be a reliable tool for non-critical components, services, or other business needs deemed not to be critical.

Supplier Maintenance Assessments

According to Kantor, an increase in supplier inspections, pursued by procurement organizations, will result in an increased likelihood of supplier's compliance to standards and subsequent improvements in productivity. Additionally, buyer behavior must align with their company's strategy for vendor management. Furthermore, customers must forge closer working relationships with their supplier base. Finally, intimate relationships with suppliers can result in risk management becoming a transparent activity.

Performing annual supplier assessments, premised on a schedule, does not make fiscal sense nor does this approach enhance supplier performance. Once supplier selection has occurred, through a well-documented supplier assessment process, organizational need and supplier performance dictates the requirement for future supplier assessments. Mayer, Nickerson, and Owan believe there is a trade-off in regards to costs associated with the inspection of a supplier's plant.

So what does Dr. D say? It really does not make good business sense to create a maintenance assessment schedule that is premised on performing on-site assessments for your entire approved supplier base, on an annual basis. This approach is fiscally prohibitive, with the costs directly proportional to the number of suppliers on your ASL. As Dr. D has stated many times; "these assessments should be driven by organizational need and risk (business risk and the actual risk of product failure)." For example, a supplier such as your sterilization provider, contract manufacturer, or metrology laboratory will probably warrant an annual on-site visit, due to the influence and importance that suppliers in these categories exude on your business. However, a machined-component supplier or injection-molding supplier (component suppliers) may require a visit once every two or three years. Bad suppliers, failing to meet expectations and requirements, place medical device organizations at risk; and should be given the boot unceremoniously. Do not waste your time throwing proverbial good money after bad. Make sure your organization has an exit strategy.

An intelligently designed questionnaire can be employed in place of an on-site visit for suppliers meeting your expectations. You may also want to consider subcontracting out the maintenance assessments to a third party auditor. One thing to remember is that the third party service provider is a contractor and must be assessed accordingly. A supplier not meeting expectations may require a simple visit to review process-specific issues. If your suppliers are evaluated annually, by competent registrars or notified bodies; the quality system aspects of their organizations should be fairly well documented (in writing remember) and robust. Selecting suppliers with quality systems approved by registrars and notified bodies will allow your organization to focus on process-related issues and drive continuous improvement projects, which add real value to an organization. Ah - yes, suppliers receiving multiple Form 483 observations or the gift of an FDA Warning Letter warrant special attention.

The Specification

So why is the specification so important? For starters, you cannot give the proverbial napkin drawing to a supplier or potential supplier and expect the supplier to meet any resemblance of quantified requirements or reasonable quality expectations, period! In fact, I dare you to give a napkin drawing to the FDA, MHLW, Health Canada, Competent Authorities in the EU, or your notified body. Besides, it is the 21st Century; and an engineering notebook is the new napkin drawing, rhetorically speaking.

A good specification not only facilitates an effective procurement process, it supports the sometimes-necessary evil known as defensive-receiving inspection and the entire 1st Article process. Additionally, a well-defined specification should employ proper dimensional-tolerancing techniques in accordance with ASME Y14.5M, when appropriate. Furthermore, the specification should contain sufficient granularity to ensure the supplier has enough technical information to manufacturer and supply a product meeting all quality and technical requirements. Secondary processes such as plating, electro-polishing, chemical-cleaning, special testing requirements, and similar subsidiary processing require consideration for inclusion into the specification. Finally, the specification should be reviewed and approved by a cross-functional team and placed under revision control, within your document control system. Why? Repeat after me, "If the specification is not documented – in writing, it does not exist." I strongly recommend attaching a copy of the specification to the contract or purchase order, prior to the issuance of these documents to your supplier. A copy of the specification should also be sent to the supplier every-single time a change order is issued. This will ensure your supplier always as the most current and hopefully, the correct revision of the specification.

Employing an effective strategy, including the implementation of three-dimensional modeling and geometric dimensioning and tolerancing early in the specification process saves money. In today's design-to-manufacture environment, drawing changes can cost anywhere from several hundred to several thousand dollars. The current model employed by most organizations is premised on: (a) recognition of need; (b) conceptual design; (c) computer aided design (CAD) with only a limited number of nominal dimensions; (d) best shot in producing samples; (e) the testing and tweaking of prototypes; and (f) feedback requiring changes to the original drawing.

Employing geometric dimensioning and tolerancing from design inception will result in manufacturing organizations circumventing potential design pitfalls early in the development phase.

Another feature, founded on a well-defined specification, is the identification of key features that can be measured by a supplier, and the statistical data provided for review, in lieu of performing defensive-receiving inspection. These same key features can be categorized within the specification as critical, major, minor, or audit. The categories drive the sampling sizes required, if defensive-receiving inspection becomes necessary. Not wanting to over-simplify the process, key features, when held within their specification limits, can be measured and the data analyzed, to gauge the overall conformance to a specification, without having to measure every feature. This data can also be employed to establish some minimum level of process capability (Ppk) by the supplier.

1st Article Inspection

Raise your hand if you think a FAI is the measuring of the initial component or first production lot. If you raised your hand, you would be incorrect, now if you actually raised your hand, please lower it, and read on. In support of establishing an effective FAI process, a supplier must be able to manufacture product in accordance with the component or procurement specification. The process commences with the supplier and the manufacturer agreeing on the data and format, completing the FAI, and then analyzing the data for accuracy and correlation. The concept of the first-article inspection has different meanings for different organizations; however, it is much more than the inspection of the first manufactured component. Additionally, it is not the intent of Dr. D to castigate ineffective FAI practices pursued by other organizations, but to bring into focus world-class practices needed to execute an effective FAI.

Prior to Dr. D's migration into the medical device world, the doctor spent several years working within the aerospace and defense industry. Similar to the medical device industry, the aerospace and defense industry is a heavily regulated industry. In fact, Dr. D strongly recommends that you find some time and actually read AS9102. AS9102 is the current aerospace standard governing FAI for the aerospace industry. One of the benefits gleaned from the employment of AS9102 is consistency in the FAI process. Initially, organizations categorized the AS9102 approach to FAI as a fiscally prohibitive approach due to the costs directly linked with the extended inspection hours associated with performing a detailed FAI. However, due to the potential for escalating costs resulting from product failure, AS9102 is a proven tool for reducing the number of product non-conformances reaching the field.

The FAI process is an integral requirement needed for material qualification and supplier certification. The FAI process consists of measuring a statistically significant sample randomly selected from each of the initial manufacturing runs (a minimum of three is recommended) provided by a supplier. Additionally, the supplier is required to execute a Gage R & R Study to support the accuracy of dimensional measurements and the effectiveness of the tools employed for the measurement process. The FAI process adheres to a predetermined sample-size requirement for all dimensional measurements premised on risk of product failure and input extracted from the design failure modes and effects analysis, (DFMEA). Finally, you, as the medical device manufacturer, must work with the supplier in the identification of characteristics to be measured, and the subsequent collection and analysis of statistical data that will be employed as a gauge for ongoing production. Remember, the expectation is that the supplier is the expert in the manufacturing of material employed in the manufacturing of finished medical devices. The supplier's expertise drives the need for the supplier to take the lead in identifying the appropriate characteristics requiring ongoing measurement and monitoring for statistical analysis.

Earlier in this chapter, I mentioned Critical (C), Major (M), Minor (m), and Audit (A) as categories for features requiring measurement/evaluation. The sample-sizes, dimensions requiring measurement, process capability requirements, etc. should be defined in advance, with supplier input/acknowledgment, and linked directly to the feature category. As criticality, premised on the DFMEA, increases, so should sample sizes for the associated feature requiring measurement. Additionally, although not a pre-requisite, I recommend designing your own FAI form. This document should be constructed so the supplier can quickly enter measurement data. Considering all of the statistical packages on the market today, such as Minitab™ (once again - not a paid spokesperson), a supplier must be able to provide accurate process capability data and attach the results to your own documentation. Once the supplier completes their FAI and provides the samples, results, statistical data, etc., you should plan to repeat the entire process internally. What, I should repeat work that has already been paid for and completed by my supplier? Yes, this is the one of the few times Dr. D finds some value in defensive-receiving inspection. It is also a sure-fire way to ensure you and your suppliers are on the same page, as ascertained through the successful correlation of the FAI results. This process also feeds nicely into the concept of SSD and the employment of SSD to reduce the defensive-receiving inspection burden.

Supplier Statistical Data (SSD)

Through the employment of an interactive approach to supplier management, with active supplier participation, tools such as the collection and analysis of measurement data can result in a reduction in the defensive-receiving inspection pursued. In conjunction with the first-article inspection process, it is a reasonable expectation that the specification creators glom the opportunity and work with the suppliers in the determination of critical features requiring measurement in support of the SSD process. Not wanting to sound like a broken record, the supplier has the capability to identify the correct dimensions needed to gage the overall effectiveness of their manufacturing processes and the sustainability of long-term process control. In fact, FAI and SSD requirements should be built into the same specification. This same specification can depict the importance of each feature (C, M, m, and A) and link criticality and risk directly to a sampling plan, aligned with the DFMEA

Each supplier selected for participation in the supplied data program should meet certain requirements prior to inclusion into this program. As a minimum, the supplier should pass an initial supplier assessment (including a review of the D & B Report), pass the FAI for the component(s) being procured, complete a supplier non-disclosure agreement, meet a pre-determined level of process capability during the first-article process, and sustain a minimum level of process capability during production. Eventually, the goal is to push the supplier toward Six-Sigma compliance, a Ppk of 2.0. Additionally, each supplier should meet the following criteria to qualify for inclusion into a SSD program.

1. The supplier and the medical device manufacturer must sign the jointly created (supplier and manufacturer input) SSD agreement that delineates the features requiring measurement and the appropriate sample sizes.

2. A minimum of number of consecutive lots (recommend at least three) must pass the appropriate defensive-receiving inspection criteria, with no defects or anomalies noted.

3. No supplier corrective action requests or similar supplier remediation activities are outstanding.

Finally, you need to ensure your suppliers and inspectors receive adequate training in support of the SSD program. The doctor has witnessed suppliers providing the wrong measurement data or supplying component lots with targeted process control limits lower than the agreed upon SSD agreement. Even worse, Dr. D has witnessed receiving inspection organizations accepting component lots premised on the availability of the SSD, without verifying the data is acceptable. Remember, SSD is ultimately a reduced approach to defensive-receiving inspection and not a paper exercise requiring the proverbial rubberstamp.

Supplier Corrective Action Requests

So, why are SCARs important? For starters, the SCAR becomes the primary vehicle for driving corrective action when issues arise with your supplier base. Remember, the FDA is concerned about the rising number of recalls premised on supplier-related issues. In the May 2007 edition of The Sheet, Kim Trautman (FDA QSR Expert) expanded on the increasing number of recalls driven by poor supplier performance. Additionally, the SCAR becomes an important metric when measuring the overall performance of your suppliers.

Now it might seem like a daunting task to issue a SCAR for every single supplier error, regardless of how benign; however, you can defend having a two-tier SCAR system. What, has the good doctor slipped off his rocker again? Seriously, an approach that I recommend is placing your SCARs into two categories. The first category is "*Response Required*" and the second category is "*For Information Only*." So what is the difference? For serious non-conformances, such as dimensional issues, repeat failures, lack of supplier responsiveness, degradation in supplier yield or performance, you are going to want detailed responses that provide insight and root-cause analysis into performance issues or non-conformances. For example, you will want the supplier to acknowledge the performance issue or non-conformance, address previous, current, and future impact from the performance issue or non-conformance, perform a detailed root-cause analysis, and very important – ensure a follow-up is performed to determine the effectiveness of all corrective actions pursued. For minor annoyances such as, the wrong quantities delivered, a torn or damaged certificates of conformance, damaged packaging not impacting the procured product, or similar non-frequent non-conformances that do not impact product performance (e.g., form, fit, or function) the "For Information Only" doubles as a nice little love letter to your supplier acknowledging that you have identified a minor issue. However, if you issue several of these love letters, to the same supplier, you just might have a significant performance problem that now requires a response.

One part of the SCAR process you should never take for granted is the follow-up / verification. Sure, your supplier is going to make an honest attempt to fix and resolve all non-conformances; however, as a medical device manufacturer it is your responsibility to verify the corrective action implemented is effective. Additionally, when employing a "Response Required" SCAR, ensure the supplier clearly understands the problem, your expectations for a solution, due date, and other relevant information. Furthermore, make sure the supplier actually receives the SCAR. If necessary, obtain a signature or some other proof of delivery. A follow-up telephone call, documented of course, is also recommended. Finally, a SCAR is a supplier metric. It should be tracked an aged accordingly, with the information presented in your management review, and the information shared with the supplier as part of their quarterly review. Some key components of the SCAR form to be considered are:

A. The SCAR tracking number;

B. The date the SCAR was issued;

C. SCAR Type (Information Only or Response Required);

D. The date the SCAR response is due;

E. The supplier name, address, point of contact, etc.;

F. The purchase order number or other relevant documentation;

G. A clear description of the non-conformance or performance issue;

H. Preventive and corrective action taken by the supplier;

I. Appropriate signatures, approvals and dates of the issuer and the supplier;

J. A section for follow-up to determine effectiveness of action pursued; and

K. Signature of approver and date SCAR was approved (or rejected).

Supplier Metrics

Providing timely and objective feedback to the supplier is an integral part of any supplier management program. Timely feedback, especially feedback relating to potential product or performance issues, requires an immediate supplier notification to ensure mitigation of risks resulting from potential non-conformances occurs. According to

Foxton, the employment of a four-step process, suitable for multiple environments, can assist in the facilitating of this feedback process. The four process phases are:

1. Pre-planning;

2. Defining and sharing of the expectations;

3. Employing recognized quality improvement techniques through the quality plans; and

4. Pursing continuous quality improvements.

According to Slobodow, Abdullah, and Babuschak the communication between the buyer and the supplier in a typical buyer-supplier relationship is absent. Additionally, Slobodow et al. believed an open and honest relationship facilitated by good communication, between the buyer and the supplier is needed. Furthermore, Slobodow et al. stated, "dual accountability between a buyer and its strategic suppliers, through tools such as a Two-Way Scorecard, is a new and tangible approach to improving supply chain relationships." Finally, the creation of a two-way scorecard is not sufficient without buy-in from senior management and cascaded down through the ranks of an organization.

One of the most important factors associated with an effective supplier management system is the ability to communicate effectively with suppliers. According to Foxton, a report card is one of the tools needed in support of effectively managing a relationship between customers and suppliers. The issuance of quarterly performance reports and the expeditious issuance of supplier corrective action requests, as appropriate, ensure suppliers receive accurate measurement guidance that accurately reflects overall supplier performance. According to Trautman in an article published in The Street, medical device manufacturers "should keep a running tally of the supplier's performance."

So what does Dr. D have to say? The doctor is a big fan of supplier corrective action and the employment of the Supplier Corrective Action Request, a.k.a., the SCAR. Supplier non-conformances are a major component and significant gage for over all supplier performance; however, they are not the only gage. Additionally, supplier yields, on-time delivery performance, responsiveness (timely response to requests), continuous improvement, value-added activities, total-cost-of-ownership, etc. can be weaved into an all-encompassing supplier report card; and yes you must ensure the supplier actually receives a copy. Depending on your organizational structure, you can decide how often to issue these report cards. In a perfect world, the data would be available real-time and on a daily basis; however, monthly would be outstanding, quarterly expected, and annually, well what is the point. As for what suppliers receive as a report card and the frequency of receipt, the decision will be premised on your organizational need and the applicable organizational procedure(s). Oh yes, before Dr. D forgets, this activity must be documented in writing because if it is not documented in writing, the event did not occur.

Purchasing Controls

According to Silva, in an interview by J. Schildhouse, "if procurement is not involved early in the process you just become the person who writes the PO." Additionally, organizational need drives the building of each business case. Furthermore, organizational buy-in allows the procurement organization to build cross-functional sourcing teams. According to Zhang, the primary objective of purchasing management is the obtainment of purchased supplies or services while sustaining price, quality, and delivery objectives. Establishing clear objectives for the purchasing organization, understanding the impact of global sourcing, and establishing strong relationships with suppliers are mandatory. In today's competitive global environment, traditional purchasing objectives require an upgrade to ensure continuous alignment with current strategic objectives. According to Buffaloe, the purchase order becomes the primary contracting document with the supplier. Within the medical device industry, if contractor or supplier provides a finished medical device, they must be managed in accordance with the Quality System Regulation. The purchase order should contain critical information such as component cost, quantity, delivery requirements, and applicable quality covenants. Additionally, the component specification, procedures for special processing steps, non-disclosure agreements, no-change agreements, and similar binding legal documents are key documents, and support the purchase order as attachments. Work authorization does not commence until completing the review of applicable agreements, signed by the appropriate level of authority, as authorized by the supplier. Finally, according to Zhenjia, overall procurement objectives must be clearly defined.

To many quality professionals, interest in developing an effective procurement organization is more of a *"velleity"* (look-it-up) than a statement of practice. However, an effective purchasing process, with competent buyers, is a supplier quality engineer's best friend. Once a supplier has been approved and added to the AVL, an organization needs a tool to obtain goods and services. That vehicle my friends, is the purchase order (PO). The PO should contain sufficient granularity to ensure the supplier has all of the necessary technical information, supply chain information, price, terms and conditions, specific quality requirements, etc. Dr. D is a strong believer of putting everything in writing and yes, I can at times sound like a broken record. For example, the PO is great;

however, a well-written supplier agreement attached to the PO, even better. The more information a supplier is provided, assuming that the information is current and accurate, the better the results. Additionally, I cannot place enough emphasis on the **NO-CHANGE AGREEMENT!** If a supplier balks at or is unwilling to sign-up to one, do not walk away, do not run away, sprint away, at God's speed. Remember folks, we are in the medical device industry; and changes require validation, regardless how benign the changes seem, just ask the FDA. Furthermore, specifications, drawings, special processes, special requirements, **SHALL** always be attached to the purchase order. Every time a change is required, a change order (revised purchase order) needs to be issued to the supplier, no exceptions, and do not forget to attach the specification / drawing with every change order. If you are a supplier, do not accept the order if all of the documentation is not attached to the PO. Are you crazy Dr. D? You want us to turn away business? No, I am not asking suppliers to turn away business; however, I am asking suppliers to hold themselves accountable for their own success. I call it being at the center of your own attention. Finally, ensure that all of your quality requirements are clearly defined. One way to accomplish this task is to insert all of the quality-specific requirements directly into the purchase order. Another way to accomplish the same task is to create a quality document that contains all of the quality requirements and assign quality codes. For example, (a) Quality Requirement Code 1A – must have an ISO 13485:2003 quality system approved by a recognized notified body, with a current certificate on file; (b) Quality Requirement Code 1B – Copy of FDA facility registration required; (c) Quality Requirement Code 1C – Certificate of Conformance required with each shipment; or (d) Quality Requirement Code 2A – No process changes or changes to material permitted. Remember, these are your codes so ensure all avenues are covered.

Takeaways

There are several takeaways from this whitepaper that should assist in helping you develop a world-class supplier management program that complies with the requirements of the QSR and ISO 13485, etc. Please keep in mind, the concept of effective supplier management is more encompassing than just supplier assessments and SCARs. In fact, purchasing, statistical concepts, 1st Articles, purchasing, purchase orders, risk, specifications, DFMEAs, and other influencers relevant to your organization's established business model must be considered. Remember, because of an increase in medical device recalls, the FDA is continuing to raise the bar in regards to supplier management and overall compliance to the QSR. That being said, Dr. D. strongly recommends the following concepts be considered when establishing a robust approach to supplier management. As a minimum, elements requiring consideration are:

1. A supplier selection process that encompasses business and product risk;

2. A requirements-driven selection process, including assessment survey (a one-shoe approach is not effective);

3. A requirement to review the D & B Report as part of the assessment process;

4. A link back to the DFMEA for determining component risk and supplier categories;

5. Supplier categories that support your organization's business model;

6. Supplier-assessment surveys tailored to specific commodities;

7. A systemic approach for pursuing supplier-maintenance assessments;

8. Robust and clear specifications;

9. A well-defined process for FAIs;

10. A program for establishing supplier statistical data;

11. A well-defined SCAR process, including a form;

12. A definition of supplier metrics to be collected, i.e., yield or on-time performance; and

13. Effective purchasing controls (purchase orders, supplier agreements, no-change agreements, and quality codes.

In reviewing these 13 elements, the key is to develop a supplier management program that is effective. There is no correct answer when creating the supplier management system; and the FDA, Competent Authorities, and Notified Bodies, are tasked with verifying compliance. Remember, compliance to regulations is mandatory, procedures are required, and documenting the results are not only required but your best defense when the agency comes knocking on your door for a friendly visit. In closing, I would like to leave you with one final thought. Regardless of the approach pursued for supplier management, product safety and efficacy is mission critical. If the finished medical device, you organization is distributing, fails to meet its specification and intended use; or even worse hurts a patient; rest assured, a visit from the FDA will be forthcoming. Finally, I recommend subscribing to The Medical Device Summit, an on-line magazine. The subscription is free and while Dr. D provides weekly advice in his blog Devine Guidance.

"Suppliers providing defective products are directly related to an increase medical device recalls!"

Management Review – The Buck Stops Here

Management Reviews

Folks, in this chapter Dr. D is going to talk about a topic that is almost never cited as a Form 483 observation or in an agency warning letter, Management Responsibility and specifically, Management Review. Frequently, the doctor likes to throw around one of his favorite terms, the Chief Jailable Officer (CJO), typically the most senior quality/regulatory person at a company. However, there can be more than one. In fact, if you are part of the executive management team, you should be orange-jumpsuit ready if you or your organization is not doing the right things. So why management review Dr. D? During a recent visit to the FDA warning letter database, the doctor came across a warning letter that cited a device manufacturer for not performing management reviews. People, holding a management review meeting is one of the most basic elements of an effective quality management system (QMS), period! If your organization is not actively pursuing management review meetings then the doctor *"importunes"* (look-it-up) you to start by holding one as soon as humanly possible. For all you CJOs that are struggling to get your management team to attend management reviews; please reinforce the requirement with your team. Feel free to share the warning letter from this chapter's guidance and remember; "The buck stops with the management team!" Enjoy.

Subpart B--Quality System Requirements

Sec. 820.20 Management responsibility.

(a) *Quality policy.* Management with executive responsibility shall establish its policy and objectives for, and commitment to, quality. Management with executive responsibility shall ensure that the quality policy is understood, implemented, and maintained at all levels of the organization.

(b) ***Organization***. Each manufacturer shall establish and maintain an adequate organizational structure to ensure that devices are designed and produced in accordance with the requirements of this part.

    (1) ***Responsibility and authority***. Each manufacturer shall establish the appropriate responsibility, authority, and interrelation of all personnel who manage, perform, and assess work affecting quality, and provide the independence and authority necessary to perform these tasks.

    (2) ***Resources.*** Each manufacturer shall provide adequate resources, including the assignment of trained personnel, for management, performance of work, and assessment activities, including internal quality audits, to meet the requirements of this part.

    (3) ***Management representative.*** Management with executive responsibility shall appoint, and document such appointment of, a member of management who, irrespective of other responsibilities, shall have established authority over and responsibility for:

        (i) Ensuring that quality system requirements are effectively established and effectively maintained in accordance with this part; and

        (ii) Reporting on the performance of the quality system to management with executive responsibility for review.

(c) ***Management review***. Management with executive responsibility shall review the suitability and effectiveness of the quality system at defined intervals and with sufficient frequency according to established procedures to ensure that the quality system satisfies the requirements of this part and the manufacturer's established quality policy and objectives. The dates and results of quality system reviews shall be documented.

(d) ***Quality planning.*** Each manufacturer shall establish a quality plan which defines the quality practices, resources, and activities relevant to devices that are designed and manufactured. The manufacturer shall establish how the requirements for quality will be met.

(e) ***Quality system procedures.*** Each manufacturer shall establish quality system

procedures and instructions. An outline of the structure of the documentation used in the

quality system shall be established where appropriate.

Warning Letter Excerpt – 09 August 2013

    Folks, as Dr. D mentioned in the introduction, management responsibility is one of the lesser cited issues by the FDA as a Form 483 observation or in a warning letter. However, that doesn't mean it is not important. In fact, management responsibility and the management review requirement are immensely important. Just in case your organization needs a friendly reminder, Dr. D has taken the liberty to share an excerpt from a recently issued warning letter.

> *"Failure of management with executive responsibility to review the suitability of the quality system at defined intervals and with sufficient frequency according to established procedures to ensure the quality system satisfies the requirements of this part, as required by 21 CFR 820.20(c). For example, your firm failed to establish management review procedures and conduct management reviews as a manufacturer of a medical device."*

Management Responsibility

From a requirements perspective, complying with management responsibility is child's play in the doctor's humble opinion. The regulation breaks management responsibility down into five buckets: (a) quality policy; (b) organization; (c) management review; (d) quality planning; and (e) quality system procedures. Considering the quality policy, organizational structure, planning, and the scripting of procedures is a given for any organization, how can management review or should Dr. D state; "lack of management review" be an issue. From an FDA's perspective, organizations do not even have to share the content of the management review meeting. All that is required is evidence of a meeting being held and an agenda. Can you say meeting sign-in sheet?

Management Review

The doctor is a big proponent of the ISO 13485:2003, Clause 5.6 for use as a blueprint for the management review process. As previously stated by the doctor, evidence of compliance to the management review requirement must be provided, upon request, when asked for by an FDA investigator. If you garner any useful information from this chapter's diatribe, please let it be that ***"establishments do not have to provide the content of management reviews to FDA!"*** If you do not believe Dr. D, the doctor suggests reading §820.180(c) (Exceptions).

> (c) *Exceptions.* ***This section does not apply to the reports required by 820.20(c) Management review,*** *820.22 Quality audits, and supplier audit reports used to meet the requirements of 820.50(a) Evaluation of suppliers, contractors, and consultants, but does apply to procedures established under these provisions. Upon request of a designated employee of FDA, an employee in management with executive responsibility shall certify in writing that the management reviews and quality audits required under this part, and supplier audits where applicable, have been performed and documented, the dates on which they were performed, and that any required corrective action has been undertaken.*

Since establishments do not have to share the contents of management review, it is incumbent among establishments to establish a sign-in sheet and an agenda that reflects management review content. Why, because if an event or activity is not documented in writing, in the eyes of our friends at the agency, it never happened. Can you say objective evidence? Since the quality system regulation does not contain much granularity around what is required to be placed into management review, the doctor strongly suggests visiting ISO 13485, Clause 5.6 and specifically 5.6.2 and 5.6.3. As a minimum, management review input should contain:

- Audit results (internal, external, and supplier);

- Customer feedback (including complaints);

- The performance of processes and results of product conformity;

- Corrective and preventive action (CAPA);

- Follow-up on activities and action items assigned during previous management reviews;

- Changes influencing the quality management system;

- Recommendations for improvement; and

- New or revised regulatory requirements.

As a minimum, the output of management review should include all decisions and

activities associated with:

- All improvements required to maintain QMS effectiveness, including supporting processes;

- Product improvements related to customer requirements;

- Assessment of resource needs; and

- A determination if quality objectives are being attained and the quality policy still relevant an applicable (as scripted) for the establishment.

Management Review Frequency

Dr. D would like to ask the readers a question. Do you know the FDA's required

frequency for management review? If your answer is annually, you would be wrong. If

your answer was semi-annually, quarterly, monthly, weekly, daily, or hourly, you would

be equally wrong. The requirement is, *"at defined intervals and with sufficient*

frequency." From the doctor's perspective, although annually usually meets the ISO

13485 requirement, holding a review once a year is not effective. Dr. D recommends

holding management review quarterly.

Takeaways

For this edition of DG, the doctor will leave the readers with three takeaways.

One – management review content <u>does not</u> need to be shared with FDA during an

inspection. In fact, it would be considered a bad practice to do so. Two – use ISO 13485,

Clauses 5.6.2 and 5.6.3 as guidance when scripting your management review procedure

and specifically review inputs and outputs. Three – As a minimum, hold management

review meetings quarterly.

"Remember, establishments do not have to share the content of management review meetings with FDA, only evidence that the meetings are being held as defined frequencies!"

Complaint Files – Stop the Complaining!

Complaint Files – Stop the Complaining

Sometimes it seems like the blasted telephone just will not stop ringing. If you work for a medical device manufacturer and are tasked with managing customer complaints, you just might want to scream. However, if the product complaints are beginning to pile up, please take notice, your customers are trying to tell you something. If you fail to address customer complaints or concerns, eventually the phone will stop ringing. Why? Well if you have to ask why, then all hope is lost. However, the doctor is obliged to provide an answer to the age-old question why. The phone will stop ringing, because your competition will be taking care of your customers. However, your organization will probably not be off the proverbial hook. The FDA may show up for a cup of coffee and an unannounced inspection in an attempt to understand what in the heck is going on with your medical device manufacturing establishment. In fact, it is the doctor's personal observation that when a device establishment is racking up large numbers of complaints, the numbers of MDRs are increasing accordingly; and that is what attracts the agency's attention. So stop complaining and enjoy this chapter's guidance; and remember, Dr. D's guidance is never marked by "*tergiversation*" (look-it-up).

Subpart M—Records

Sec. 820.198 Complaint files

(a) Each manufacturer shall maintain complaint files. Each manufacturer shall establish and maintain procedures for receiving, reviewing, and evaluating complaints by a formally designated unit. Such procedures shall ensure that:

(1) All complaints are processed in a uniform and timely manner;

(2) Oral complaints are documented upon receipt; and

(3) Complaints are evaluated to determine whether the complaint represents an event which is required to be reported to FDA under part 803 of this chapter, Medical Device Reporting.

(b) Each manufacturer shall review and evaluate all complaints to determine whether an investigation is necessary. When no investigation is made, the manufacturer shall maintain a record that includes the reason no investigation was made and the name of the individual responsible for the decision not to investigate.

(c) Any complaint involving the possible failure of a device, labeling, or packaging to meet any of its specifications shall be reviewed, evaluated, and investigated, unless such investigation has already been performed for a similar complaint and another investigation is not necessary.

(d) Any complaint that represents an event which must be reported to FDA under part 803 of this chapter shall be promptly reviewed, evaluated, and investigated by a designated individual(s) and shall be maintained in a separate portion of the complaint files or otherwise clearly identified. In addition to the information required by 820.198(e), records of investigation under this paragraph shall include a determination of:

(1) Whether the device failed to meet specifications;

(2) Whether the device was being used for treatment or diagnosis; and

(3) The relationship, if any, of the device to the reported incident or adverse event.

(e) When an investigation is made under this section, a record of the investigation shall be maintained by the formally designated unit identified in paragraph (a) of this section. The record of investigation shall include:

(1) The name of the device;

(2) The date the complaint was received;

(3) Any device identification(s) and control number(s) used;

(4) The name, address, and phone number of the complainant;

(5) The nature and details of the complaint;

(6) The dates and results of the investigation;

(7) Any corrective action taken; and

(8) Any reply to the complainant.

(f) When the manufacturer's formally designated complaint unit is located at a site separate from the manufacturing establishment, the investigated complaint(s) and the record(s) of investigation shall be reasonably accessible to the manufacturing establishment.

(g) If a manufacturer's formally designated complaint unit is located outside of the United States, records required by this section shall be reasonably accessible in the United States at either:

(1) A location in the United States where the manufacturer's records are regularly kept; or

(2) The location of the initial distributor.

Complaints

The doctor is going to begin by stating; "You need to script a procedure that addresses §820.198;" however, do not stop there. The complaint procedure also needs to link to Medical Device Reports (MDR) and the need to file MDRs within five or 30-days. In fact, the complaint management procedure should have a direct link to whatever document your organization employs for 21 CFR, Part 803, Medical Device Reporting. If your establishment is selling product into the European Union (EU), then a link to the requirements delineated within MEDDEV 2.12-1, Revision 8, Guidelines on a Medical Devices Vigilance System, is also warranted. If you choose to do so, you can make one cohesive complaint management SOP that covers all bases. However, as your organization progresses into multiple markets, the requirements will start to multiply, as well. The doctor is not going to waste the time of the readers by reviewing all of the tiny nuances needing to be addressed in a SOP. You can purchase Devine Guidance for

Complying with the FDA's QSR from Amazon.com – (http://www.amazon.com/Devine-Guidance-Complying-Quality-Regulation/dp/1466358769/ref=sr_1_1?s=books&ie=UTF8&qid=1380197472&sr=1-1&keywords=devine+guidance). However, Dr. D is going to address the salient requirements that a complaint management procedure needs to encompass.

Essential Elements of a Complaint Management SOP

So what are the essential elements of complaint management? Once the SOP has been scripted, it starts with training. Obviously, the in-house folks tasked with managing complaints need to be trained. However, do not forget about the front-line employees, the sales force. Regardless of how benign a customer complaint might appear to be, it needs to be reported. For example, if a physician puts an itsy-bitsy-tiny hole in a surgical glove because of a sharp edge on a catheter handle, that is a complaint. Is it going to be an MDR, probably not? If a device fails to work out of the box it is going to be a complaint. Is it going to be an MDR, probably not? If a member of your sales team is reading a medical journal and stumbles upon an article that "*disparages*" (look-it-up) on of your organization's medical devices, that my friends is a reportable complaint. Is it going to be an MDR? It depends and Dr. D is not talking about adult diapers. The need to report will be premised on the outcome of the investigation.

That being said, essential elements of a complaint management SOP are:

- Collecting basic complaint information (read §820.198 for specifics);
- Recovering the device that the complaint is premised on;
- Decontaminating the device, if it has been used;
- Performing a thorough **root cause investigation**;

- Employing a decision tree to determine if the complaint is reportable as and MDR in the United States (reference Part 803); a vigilance report in the EU (reference MEDDEV 2.12-1); or reportable elsewhere;

- If deemed necessary and appropriate, open a Corrective Action in your CAPA System to address and correct the complaint;

- Make sure all complaints are reviewed and approved by a person with a clinical/medical background (note: should be a physician, nurse practitioner, or registered nurse); and

- Send a follow-up letter to the complainant, if one is requested (a well-worded professional response always a nice gesture).

Takeaways

For this chapter's guidance, the doctor will leave the readers with five takeaways. One – if you receive a complaint, consider it valuable feedback from your customer. They are reaching out to your organization. Two – always perform an in-depth failure investigation. Three – not all complaints are required to be reported as MDRs; however, you darn well better make sure that the complaints that rate as MDRs are reported. Four – ensure an individual with a clinical/medical background reviews and approves all complaints. Five – if your organization fails to correct the issues associated with a complaint, trust the doctor when I say; "Your competition will gladly help your customers move their business!"

If a device fails to work out of the box it is going to be a complaint!

Purchasing Controls –
Where's the Purchase Order?

Purchasing Controls – Where's the Purchase Order?

Folks, one of the issues that Dr. D continues to see medical device establishment struggle with is implementing effective controls. In fact, if you visit the FDA's Enforcement Page; you will quickly being able to ascertain that the agency has concerns over industry's compliance with 21 CFR, Part 820.50 (Purchasing Controls). For this chapter, the doctor is going to focus on the purchasing piece, a.k.a., *"purchasing data"* and not the supplier management aspect of purchasing controls, even though the *"evaluation of suppliers, contractors, and consultants"* is a salient component of *"purchasing controls."* Besides, instead of hurling disparaging remarks at the supplier quality engineers, Dr. D would like to enlighten the procurement folks for a change. As one of the doctor's favorite comedians is always saying (Carlos Mencia); "It's just your turn, so just take it!" As the frequent readers of the doctor's tirades know, the doctor never attempts to be too showy or *"ostentatious"* (look-it-up) with his writing. The doctor likes to provide guidance with an edge. Enjoy!

Subpart E—Purchasing Controls

Sec. 820.50 Purchasing controls.

Each manufacturer shall establish and maintain procedures to ensure that all purchased or otherwise received product and services conform to specified requirements.

(a) *Evaluation of suppliers, contractors, and consultants.* Each manufacturer shall establish and maintain the requirements, including quality requirements, that must be met by suppliers, contractors, and consultants. Each manufacturer shall:

(1) Evaluate and select potential suppliers, contractors, and consultants on the basis of their ability to meet specified requirements, including quality requirements. The evaluation shall be documented.

(2) Define the type and extent of control to be exercised over the product, services, suppliers, contractors, and consultants, based on the evaluation results.

(3) Establish and maintain records of acceptable suppliers, contractors, and consultants.

(b) *Purchasing data.* Each manufacturer shall establish and maintain data that clearly describe or reference the specified requirements, including quality requirements, for purchased or otherwise received product and services. Purchasing documents shall include, where possible, an agreement that the suppliers, contractors, and consultants agree to notify the manufacturer of changes in the product or service so that manufacturers may determine whether the changes may affect the quality of a finished device. Purchasing data shall be approved in accordance with 820.40.

Where's the Purchase Order?

Let the doctor begin by stating, I am probably one of the worst violators when it comes to obtaining a purchase order prior to commencing work for the doctor's clients. Dr. D is usually happy with a signed statement of work (SOW). Since the SOWs are extremely prescriptive, this is probably not an issue. Dr. D is only attempting to make life a bit easier for the doctor's clients. However, a purchase order is always the preferred path. In fact, a purchase order that delineates sufficient information to ensure the correct goods and services are purchased needs to be a fundamental requirement. Additionally, any and all supporting documentation such as drawings, specifications, standards, etc. should be referenced in the purchase order and sent to the **approved supplier** as an attachment to the purchase order. Furthermore, if a drawing, specification, or standard changes, a change order with the new/revised documentation should be sent to the **approved supplier**. Finally, best practice is to have a signed quality agreement with critical suppliers. Obviously, the legal folks always want to put their stamp of approval on such documents, but generic ones are easily obtained off the Internet that delineate the basic requirements and set essential expectations for suppliers.

Can You Say Form 483 Observation?

One of the issues Dr. D typically sees when performing client internal and supplier audits is a lack of control over the issuance of purchase orders. For example, in an R & D environment, an engineer or even a buyer will get on the phone and call in an order for 100 machined components for a new catheter from ACME Machining (fictitious name). ACME is not on the Approved Supplier's List, an unreleased drawing is sent to ACME, no formal purchase order is issued, just a number. So guess what happened next? The parts are shipped to the medical device manufacturer and they sit on the receiving dock because there is no purchase order to receive the parts against. The buyer finally creates the purchase order and the parts find their way into incoming inspection. The quality folks do the right thing and reject the parts for not having a released drawing and being procured from a supplier not listed on the ASL. Weeks later, the engineer finally gets the parts. Unfortunately, this process continues to repeat itself and low and behold FDA shows up for a cup of coffee and an inspection. While using the infamous CAPA plus one technique the FDA investigator selects nonconforming material. While reviewing the nonconforming material reports the investigator quickly comes to the conclusion that purchasing is procuring material from unapproved suppliers and without the proper purchasing documentation. Can you say Form 483 observation? Now granted, you are probably laughing and saying to yourselves, Dr. D that never happens. If you believe that, the doctor just purchased the old Bay Bridge and is offering it up for sale.

Don't Forget About the No-Change Agreements

Now Dr. D knows that FDA does not like surprises and neither should you. The doctor has seen far too many recalls because a supplier has suffered a major brain fart and forgot to notify the device manufacturer of a tiny little change, like we changed the raw material from polycarbonate to ABS, our bad! If a valid no-change agreement is in place and supported by a quality agreement or similar type of contract then the device manufacturer will probably have some legal recourse. Once again, make sure legal blesses the no-change agreement. If you do not have a legal group, you can have Dr. D bless it.

Incoming Inspection, a Necessary Evil

As many of the readers already know, Dr. D is not a big proponent of incoming inspection. Device manufacturers pay good money for their services and materials. Considering the money being spent, the expectation should be that everything procured is conforming to requirements, all of the time, every time. Unfortunately, that type of medical device utopia still does not exist, thanks in part to Mr. Murphy being alive and well in the medical device industry. That being said, the doctor believes that inspection should be employed intelligently and sparingly. Please feel free to put the onus on your suppliers through supplied data and similar statistical programs.

Takeaways

For this chapter's guidance the doctor will leave the readers with three takeaways. One – always take the time and create a purchase order. Two – only place purchase orders with suppliers list on the ASL. Three – only use released drawings to purchase materials. If you feel the need for speed your organization can differentiate developmental drawings versus production through the use of numeric revisions for development and alpha revisions for production. Four – always have quality agreements and no-change agreements with your key suppliers. Five – unfortunately incoming inspection is a necessary evil, thanks to Mr. Murphy, so use it wisely.

Any and all supporting documentation such as drawings, specifications, standards, etc. should be referenced in the purchase order and sent to the approved supplier as an attachment to the purchase order!

Training – Is that Really Necessary?

Training – is that Really Necessary?

Man, does Dr. D love having Internet access on airplanes. During a recent flight from Dallas to San Jose, the doctor was able to find time to traverse the FDA's enforcement page and came upon a fairly long and terse warning letter issued to a device establishment in Northern California. In fact, the fifteen (15) – yes that is one-five observations noted in one warning letter make it one of the most substantial letters the doctor has read in some time. Now Dr. D is not going to debate the merits of such a warning letter, especially where a device establishment is literally roasted by the agency. However, one observation, **_Training_**, the doctor finds particularly disturbing. Folks, training is one of those fundamental requirements that influence all aspects of the Quality Management System (QMS). That being said, the doctor will expand upon the virtues associated with establishing an effective training program for this chapter's guidance. For those frequent readers of Devine Guidance, please remember that Dr. D receives no **_"pecuniary"_** (look-it-up) compensation for his weekly tirades. The doctor's writing is driven by a labor of love and to teach readers about the need for complying with quality, regulatory, and statutory requirements, while gaining a loyal customer and fan base. Enjoy.

Warning Letter

As stated in the intro of this chapter's guidance, receiving a warning that contains fifteen (15) Form 483 observations is quite a feat; however, it is by no means a record. Since you or the doctor was not in attendance at this inspection what is lost in translation is the interaction between the FDA investigator and the staff of the offending establishment. One thing is for sure though; this inspection did not go well. In fact, premised on the outcome documented in the warning letter, the inspection did not go well indeed.

Warning Letter Excerpt – 20 September 2013

*Failure to establish procedures for identifying training needs and ensure that all personnel are trained to adequately perform their assigned responsibilities, as required by 21 CFR 820.25(b). For example, your firm's Risk Management procedure, SOP-0017 Version 4.0, states, "Persons performing risk management tasks shall have the knowledge and experience appropriate to the tasks assigned to them. Records of Qualifications shall be retained in the employee's Training File per SOP-0004, Training." During the inspection, the FDA investigator requested training documents for **(b)(4)** individuals who were involved in the risk analysis process. Your firm could not provide any training documentation for one of the individuals and provided a certificate titled, "FDA QSR/GMP & Inspections 2009" and associated test records for the second individual. Review of these documents revealed that they did not address risk analysis techniques.*

We have reviewed your response and have concluded that it is inadequate. Your firm updated its Risk Management procedure, SOP-0017, to Version 5.0, which now states, "Persons performing risk management tasks shall have the knowledge and experience appropriate to the tasks assigned to them. Persons should have knowledge of ISO 14971. Records of Qualifications shall be retained in the employee's Training File per SOP-0004, Training." However, your firm did not provide evidence demonstrating that it has planned, initiated or completed training of appropriate personnel to ISO-14971. Finally, your firm did not provide evidence demonstrating that personnel responsible for determining employee training needs were trained on the additional training requirement stated in the updated SOP-0017, Version 5.0.

Subpart B – Quality System Requirements

Sec. 820.25 Personnel

(a) *General.* Each manufacturer shall have sufficient personnel with the necessary education, background, training, and experience to assure that all activities required by this part are correctly performed.

(b) *Training.* Each manufacturer shall establish procedures for identifying training needs and ensure that all personnel are trained to adequately perform their assigned responsibilities. Training shall be documented.

(1) As part of their training, personnel shall be made aware of device defects which may occur from the improper performance of their specific jobs.

(2) Personnel who perform verification and validation activities shall be made aware of defects and errors that may be encountered as part of their job functions.

Training – Basic Requirements

For starters, §820.25 requires that *"sufficient personnel with the necessary education, background, training, and experience"* are available to support the operations of a medical device establishment. In short, it becomes a nearly *"insurmountable"* (look-it-up) task to train individuals that lack appropriate education, background, and experience to work in the medical device industry. For example, if the device establishment needs auditors, internal or supplier, good luck with hiring short-order cooks to fill the role. In fact, ISO 9001:2008, ISO 13485:2003, and ISO 13485:2012 are pretty explicit when dictating that auditors need to meet ISO 19011 requirements. That being said, a device establishment's best policy should be to only hire intelligent individuals with appropriate levels of education, background, training, and experience. However, please keep in mind individuals from other highly regulated industries such as pharmaceutical or aerospace and defense make fine candidates as well.

Training Program

Dr. D will start this paragraph off with a broken-record comment; "You need to have a **well-written procedure** that clearly delineates the requirements for the training program!" All employees, from the janitor to the Chief Jailable Officer (CJO) must be appropriately trained to execute their duties. For example, every-single member of an organization should receive training to the QMS, Quality Policy, and Quality Objectives.

This training needs to be documented. Why? Because if an event or activity is not documented in writing, in the eyes of FDA, it never occurred.

Additionally, the QSR is very clear in regards to: (a) ensuring personnel are made aware of device defects; (b) personnel tasked with executing verification and validation issues are made aware of defects and errors associated with executing their job function. For operators and inspectors, it is imperative that their training occur in the manufacturing environment. Supervisors and trainers must take responsibility for their direct reports and ensure their personnel are adequately trained and the training documented, **in writing!** In some instances, some level of comprehension will be required by operators and inspectors, so tests premised on practical application of job skills, after training, is probably a good idea to pursue. For exempt employees, self-training is always a viable option, providing the training is documented, **in writing!**

Furthermore, training of contractors and consultants is also a salient requirement. For example, if you decide to hire Dr. D or a member of my staff to perform internal audits, Dr. D and members of his team must be trained to your procedures, as applicable. Training to your SOPs for Internal Audits, Gowning, and other relevant procedures will be required and evidence of the training documented, **in writing!**

Finally, when FDA knocks on the front door for a cup of coffee and an inspection, do not forget that FDA requires training too! The investigator will need to be trained to such minor little things like gowning to enter the cleanroom and appropriate safety procedures such as the need to wear protective eyewear. Guess what? This training must be documented, **in writing!**

Takeaways

For this chapter's guidance the doctor will leave the readers with four takeaways. One – medical device establishments must have a well-written procedure that delineates all of the fundamental requirements for a training program. Two – being able to successfully train individuals begins with the hiring of individuals that possess *"the necessary education, background, training, and experience."* Three – remember consultants, contractors and FDA investigators require some level of training to work in a medical device establishment. Four – all training must be documented, **in writing!**

"When FDA knocks on the front door for a cup of coffee and an inspection, do not forget that FDA requires training too!"

Environmental Controls

Environmental Controls – You Need to Keep Records

Dr. D spends a bunch of time in the air flying around the country and on the road playing

road warrior. On a positive note, that gives the doctor plenty of time for drinking and

thinking. That being said, this chapter's guidance is also premised on one of the doctor's

visits to the FDA's enforcement page, during a long flight, and the opportunity to traverse

the warning letters for weekly cannon fodder. For this chapter's guidance, the doctor

came across another interesting violation of the QSR, environmental controls. If a

medical device establishment is manufacturing sterile medical devices, Dr. D is not sure

how environmental monitoring and the calibration and servicing of environmental control

systems are not part of the product realization equation. For you non ISO 13485-types,

that means manufacturing. In fact, the doctor *"asseverates"* (look-it-up) that controlled

environments must always be monitored and the results recorded as objective evidence of

compliance. If objective evidence is not recorded, than in the eyes of FDA, the event or

activity never occurred. Before jumping into this chapter's guidance, if you are your

organization's Chief Jailable Officer (CJO), then you know how much fun it is sitting

across from an FDA investigator without objective evidence of compliance. Enjoy!

Warning Letter

This chapter's warning letter was issued to a Chinese company that manufactures

catheter insertion kits, blood piercing devices, and surgical forceps. Clearly these devices

are sterile and the expectation is that they are being manufactured in a controlled

environment. However, without written procedures that define the controls such as

temperature, humidity, positive pressure, particulate counts, acceptable-levels of biocontamination (including action and alert limits), servicing of HEPA filtration systems, servicing of air handler units, and the calibration of measuring and monitoring equipment, then there is zero chance of being able to claim compliance in the eyes of FDA. The warning letter excerpt presented in this chapter's guidance was their reward as a result of a less than stellar inspection.

Warning Letter Excerpt – 19 September 2013

Failure to establish and maintain procedures to control environmental conditions that could reasonably be expected to have an adverse effect on product quality and failure to periodically inspect environmental control systems to verify that the system is adequate and functioning properly, as required by 21 CFR 820.70(c). For example, (b)(4) results for the (b)(4) area were not documented from February 2013 through June 2013.

Subpart G – Production and Process Controls

Sec. 820.70(c) Environmental Control

(c) Environmental control. Where environmental conditions could reasonably be expected to have an adverse effect on product quality, the manufacturer shall establish and maintain procedures to adequately control these environmental conditions. Environmental control system(s) shall be periodically inspected to verify that the system, including necessary equipment, is adequate and functioning properly. These activities shall be documented and reviewed.

Environmental Control – Basic Requirements

For this chapter's guidance, the doctor will be brief. Dr. D strongly recommends the process commence with the scripting of a series of Standard Operating Procedures (SOPs). The doctor recommends that you consider the following SOPs or ensure that these requirements are addressed in existing SOPs and/or work instructions:

- A procedure for gowning and hygiene of personnel appropriate for clean room (controlled environment) entry;

- An environmental controls procedure that delineates the requirements for monitoring and recording of temperature, RH, airborne particulate counts; and work-surface contamination limits (number of colony forming units – CFUs);

- A procedure for product cleanliness;

- Requirements for packaging soon-to-be sterile medical devices in a controlled environment; and

- Validation(s) to support the controlled environment capable of providing stable and repeatable results.

Additionally, the doctor strongly recommends the use of qualified suppliers, to perform all of the testing, maintenance, and validation activities, if the decision is made to outsource this work. Can you say ISO/IEC 17025:2005? There are many reputable firms available that can validate the environmental operating conditions associated with your controlled environment and keep it humming along, well below your specified alert limits (hopefully).

Recommended Standards

The best advice the doctor can offer in regards to standard utilization is the ISO 14644 series of standards. As a minimum, Dr. D recommends that the following ISO standards be considered and applied:

- ISO 14644-1:1999 (Clean Rooms and Associated Controlled Environments – Part 1: Classification of Air Cleanliness);

- ISO 14644-2:2000 (Clean Rooms and Associated Controlled Environments – Part 2: Specification for Testing and Monitoring to Prove Continued Compliance with ISO 14644-1); and

- ISO 14644-3:2005 (Clean Rooms and Associated Controlled Environments – Part 3: Test Methods).

If your organization employs compressed air, then ISO 8573-1:2010 (Compressed Air – Part 1: Contaminants and Purity Classes) should be considered. FYI – your notified body is going to ask to see compliance to ISO 8573-1, so it is better to be prepared.

Takeaways

For this chapter's guidance Dr. D will leave the readers with four takeaways. One – Compliance begins with the scripting of well-written procedures. Two – The ISO 14644 series of standards are available to help guide organizations with clear and concise requirements for clean rooms (controlled environments). Three – Always select a qualified organization for the initial validation and subsequent testing of the controlled environment. Four – Just in case you haven't figure it out yet, documented records/results for the monitoring of a controlled environment is a salient requirement for FDA.

"Without written procedures that define basic environmental controls, there is zero chance of being able to claim compliance in the eyes of FDA!"

Epilogue

Epilogue

Regardless of manufacturing and selling products into the United States market or anywhere else in the world, it is all about compliance. Device manufacturers are expected to have a documented Quality Management System and the system adequately supported by procedures, forms, work instructions, etc. When device establishments take short cuts, that is where they run into trouble. In the United States, because of the way information is disseminated on the FDA's website, there is no hiding from the truth. If a device establishment fails to comply with the Quality System Regulations and the agency determines the violations are egregious, then warning letters and other appropriate regulatory actions are going to be pursued. Please, **<u>do not be</u>** that offending device establishment that runs afoul of FDA or places their CJO in jeopardy of wearing that bright-orange jumpsuit. That being said, the doctor would like to personally thank all of the readers of Dr. D's fifth book. Without you, there would be no Devine Guidance, at least from a medical device perspective. Please stay-tuned for the next book "Close only counts in Chinese checkers and hand grenades" – just kidding, cheers from Dr. D and best wishes for continued professional success.

"Dr. D"

References

References

Buffaloe, V. (2006). Outsourcing and the quality system. *Biomedical Engineering & Technology, 40*(4). Retrieved January 4, 2007, from http://proquest.umi.com

Chase, N. (1999, October). Reports standardize receiving inspection. *Quality, 38*(6).

Code of Federal Regulation. (2013, April) *Title 21 Part 807: Establishment registration and device listing for manufacturers and initial importers of devices.* Washington, D.C.: U.S. Government Printing Office.

Code of Federal Regulation. (2013, April). *Title 21 Part 814: Premarket approval of medical devices.* Washington, D.C.: U. S. Government Printing Office.

Code of Federal Regulation. (2013, April). *Title 21 Part 820: Quality system regulation.* Washington, D.C.: U. S. Government Printing Office.

Cooper, R. & Fleder, J. (2005). *Responding* to a form 483 or warning letter: A practical guide. *Food and Drug Law Journal, 60*(4).

Devine, C. (2011). *Devine guidance for complying with the FDA's quality system regulation – 21 CFR, Part 820.* Charleston, SC: Amazon.

Devine, C. (2012). *Devine guidance for complying with the European medical device directive – MDD.* Charleston, SC: Amazon.

Devine, C. (2011). *White paper – effective supplier management in support of the medical device industry.*

Devine, C. (2012). *Devine guidance for complying with the European in-vitro diagnostic directive – IVDD.* Charleston, SC: Amazon.

Devine, C. (2012). *Devine Guidance series on complying with the IVDD.* Published in The Medical Device Summit. http://medicaldevicesummit.com

Devine, C. (2011). *Devine Guidance series on complying with the MDD.* Published in The Medical Device Summit. http://medicaldevicesummit.com

Dimensioning and tolerancing. (1994). *American Society of Mechanical Engineers ASME Y14.5M-1994.* New York, NY.

EN ISO 13485:2012. (2012, February). *Medical devices – quality management systems – requirements for regulatory purposes (EN ISO 13485:2012).*

FDA Guidance Document (2013, July). *Definition of Seizure.* Retrieved July 18, 2013, from http://www.fda.gov/MedicalDevices/DeviceRegulationandGuidance/GuidanceDocuments/ucm094529.htm#seizure

FDA Seizes All Medical Products From N.J. Device Manufacturer for Significant Manufacturing Violations. (2007, April). FDA Website. Retrieved July 18, 2013, from http://www.fda.gov/NewsEvents/Newsroom/PressAnnouncements/2007/ucm108893.htm

FDA - U.S. Food and Drug Administration Website. (2013). Warning letters. Retrieved March 29, 2013, from http://www.fda.gov/ICECI/EnforcementActions/WarningLetters/

FDA - U.S. Food and Drug Administration Website. (2013, June). Warning letters. Retrieved July 27, 2013, from http://www.fda.gov/ICECI/EnforcementActions/WarningLetters/2013/ucm359625.htm

Final rule – cGMP requirements for combination products. (2013, January). FDA website. Retrieved January 25, 2013, from *https://www.federalregister.gov/articles/2013/01/22/2013-01068/current-good-manufacturing-practice-requirements-for-combination-products*

Food and drug administration safety and innovation act (FDASIA). (2012, July). FDA Website. Retrieved April 20, 2013, from http://www.fda.gov/RegulatoryInformation/Legislation/FederalFoodDrugandCosmeticActFDCAct/SignificantAmendmentstotheFDCAct/FDASIA/ucm20027187.htm

Foster, M. (2003, August). 3-D and G D & T takes a concept to production. *Quality, 42*(8). Retrieved November 3, 2008, from http://proquest.umi.com

Foxton, J. (1996). Negotiating quality through customer communications. *Managing Service Quality, 6*(5). Retrieved November 5, 2008, from http://proquest.umi.com

Ghinato, P. (1998, August). Quality control methods: towards modern approaches through well-established principles. *Total Quality Management, 9*(6).

Investigations operations manual. (2013). Chapter 5 Establishment Inspections. Retrieved September 8, 2013, from http://www.fda.gov/downloads/ICECI/Inspections/IOM/UCM150576.pdf

ISO 8573-1:2010. (2010). *Compressed air – part 1: Contaminants and purity classes.*

ISO 9001:2008 (2008, November). *Quality management system- requirements (ISO 9001:2008).*

ISO 19011:2011. (2011, November). *Guidelines for quality and/or environmental management systems auditing (ISO 19011:2011).*

ISO 11135-1:2007. (2007, May). *Sterilization of healthcare products – Ethylene oxide – Part 1: Requirements for development and routine control of a sterilization process for medical devices.*

ISO 11137-1:2006. (2006, April). *Sterilization of healthcare products – Radiation – Part 1: Requirements for development, validation and routine control of a sterilization process for medical devices.*

ISO 13485:2003. (2004, February). *Medical devices – quality management systems – requirements for regulatory purposes (ISO 13485:2003).*

ISO 14644-1:1999. (1999). *Clean rooms and associated controlled environments – Part 1: Classification of air cleanliness.*

ISO 14644-2:2000. (2000). *Clean rooms and associated controlled environments – Part 2: Specification for testing and monitoring to prove continued compliance with ISO 14644-1.*

ISO 14644-3:2005. (2005). *Clean rooms and associated controlled environments – Part 3: Test methods.*

ISTA. (2011, February). International Safe Transit Association. Retrieved February 7, 2011, from http://www.ista.org/

Kanter, J. (2008, June). Audits crucial to supplier wellbeing. *Supply Management, 13*(12). Retrieved November 13, 2008, from http://proquest.umi.com

Lookabaugh, M. (2006, May). *Responding to FDA 483s and warning letters – presentation to Parenteral Drug Association.* Parexel Consulting. Lowell, MA.

Mayer, K. J., Nickerson, J. A., & Owan, H. (2004, August). *Are* supply and plant inspections complements or substitutes – a strategic and operational assessment of inspection practices in biotechnology. *Management Science, 50*(8).

MEDDEV 2.12-1, Revision 7. (2012, March). Guidelines on a medical device vigilance system. Retrieved September 26, 2013, from http://www.obelis.net/docs/Guidelines_MEDDEV_212-1_rev7_march_2012.pdf

Medical device establishment registration and listing - notice of changes for FY 2013. (2012, August). FDA Website. Retrieved April 20, 2013, from http://www.fda.gov/MedicalDevices/ResourcesforYou/Industry/ucm314844.htm

Morris, R. (2007, July). Enhance first article inspection. *Quality, 46*(7).

Poor supplier control causing recalls, FDA says; contract is key to success. (2007, May). *The Sheet – Medical Device Quality Control, 11*(6). Danvers, MA.

Process capability and performance. (2007). *MiC quality six sigma glossary.* Retrieved May 4, 2007, from http://www.micquality.com

Rossetti, A. (2008, December). *Shelhigh: anatomy of an FDA medical device product seizure.* The Legal Examiner. Retrieved July 18, 2013, from http://westpalmbeach.legalexaminer.com/medical-devices-implants/shelhigh-anatomy-of-an-fda-medical-device-products-seizure/

Schildhouse, J. (2005, summer). An interview with Sarmento Silva. *Journal of Supply Chain Management, 41*(3). Retrieved November 4, 2008, from http://proquest.umi.com

Slobodow, B., Abdullah, O., & Babuschak, C. (2008). When supplier partnerships aren't. *MIT Sloan Management Review, 49*(2).

Zhang, Z. (2008, June). Literature review of purchasing management in service industry. *Management Science and Engineering, 2*(2).

Zhenjia, Z. (2008, June). Literature review of purchasing management in service industry. *Management Science and Engineering 2*(2).

Index

Index

CPSIA information can be obtained
at www.ICGtesting.com
Printed in the USA
LVHW060011300121
677862LV00009B/611